THE SKILFUL PATHOLOGIST

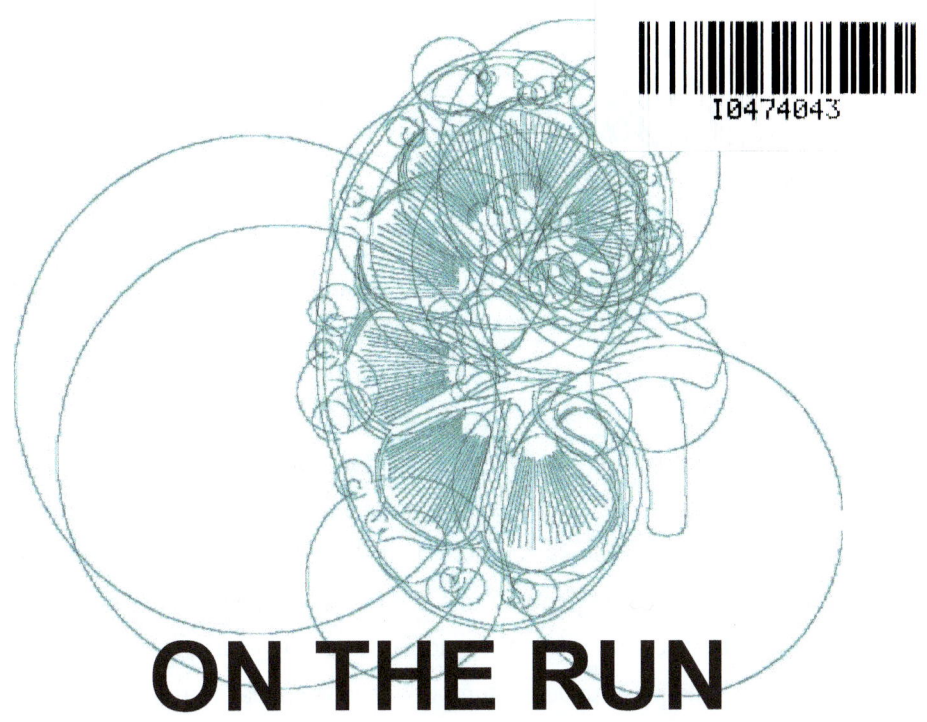

ON THE RUN

STAGING AND GRADING
OF CANCER AND NON-CANCER
IN PATHOLOGY

2021

Prof. Osama Sharaf Eldin, PhD, FRCPath

ISBN: 978-1-4710-4078-8

Dedication

I dedicate this book to the soul of my father, to my mother, to my lovely wife and to the new comer to my family, princess Lara

Preface

Staging and grading of cancer (malignant tumours) and the accuracy of allocation a certain tumour a proper stage and grade requires experience and mindful examination of tumour tissue both macroscopically (grossly) and microscopically with good use of measurements. The pathologist should be equipped by a lot of anatomical, radiological and clinical data. Staging and grading of patient's tumour tissue is crucial in further treatment either surgically or non-surgically using chemotherapy, radiotherapy or more advanced treatments including immune modulation therapies and genetic-related new treatments to approach cure or control of tumour growth and minimise patient's mortality and morbidity. In this book I tried to simplify the hugely complex pathological staging system of TNM and tumour grading, aiming at giving the reader an easy tool to apply the most up to date staging and grading without need to read complex textbooks. Non-neoplastic diseases Staging and grading are also added.

Osama Sharaf Eldin, Northern Ireland, UK, 2021.

ABBREVIATIONS:

CIS: carcinoma in situ (non-invasive carcinoma with intact basement membrane). CIS includes:
- AIN: anal intraepithelial neoplasia
- Bowen's disease: skin
- BilIN: biliary intraepithelial neoplasia
- cGIN, glandular, cervix
- CIN: cervical intraepithelial neoplasia
- CINIII, squamous cervix
- DCIS: Ductal carcinoma in situ, breast
- DIPNIC: neuroendocrine lung
- EIN: endometrial intraepithelial neoplasia and SEIC, serous endometrial intraepithelial carcinoma.
- GCNIS, germ cell neoplasia in situ, testis
- HG urothelial carcinoma in situ
- HGPIN: high grade prostatic intraepithelial neoplasia
- HSIL: high grade squamous intraepithelial lesion
- Insitu melanoma and lentigo maligna
- Intraductal carcinoma of the prostate
- LAMN: low grade appendiceal mucinous neoplasm
- LCIS: lobular carcinoma in situ
- Paget's (mammary and extramammary)
- PanIN: pancreatic intraepithelial neoplasia
- PeIN: penile intraepithelial neoplasia
- PIN: prostatic intraepithelial neoplasia
- STIC: serous tubal intraepithelial carcinoma
- VAIN: vaginal intraepithelial neoplasia
- VIN: vulvar intraepithelial neoplasia

(i): LN metastasis detected by IHC only, important in breast
(m): multiple tumours in tumour stage
(mi): micro-invasion in tumour stage or micromets in Nodal stage
Adca: adenocarcinoma
BM: basement membrane
bilat: bilateral
bx: biopsy
CT: connective tissue
CRC: colorectal carcinoma
c: clinical
contra: contralateral (opposite side)
DDx: differential diagnosis
DOI: Depth of invasion
Dx: diagnosis
EMVI: extramural vascular invasion
ENE: extra nodal extension
GB: gall bladder

HCC: hepatocellular carcinoma
Hx: history
IDC: invasive ductal carcinoma, breast
IHC: immunohistochemistry
inv: invasion
ipsi: ipsilateral (same side)
ITC: isolated tumour cells
LN: Lymph node
LVI: lymphovascular space invasion-tumour emboli
SC: subcutaneous tissue
epid: epidermis or epididymis (based on context)
 Mets: metastasis
MM: muscularis mucosa
MP: muscularis propria
n: nerve
neg (-): negative
NET: neuroendocrine tumour
NSCC: non-small cell carcinoma
OPC: oropharyngeal cancer
p: pathological
Pn: perineural invasion
pos (+): positive
R: margin
r: recurrence
RCC: renal cell carcinoma
S: serum tumour markers (from S0-normal to S3)
SCC: squamous cell carcinoma
SLNB or (sn): sentinel LN Bx
SM: submucosa
SS: subserosa
SV : seminal vesicle
T: tumour
Tx: treatment
UB: urinary bladder
unilat: unilateral
y: therapy

#Facebook:
Histopathology and Cytopathology Consultancy Group
Global Pathologists Group
Dr Osama Sharaf Eldin (page)
osamasha@gmail.com

I. PATHOLOGICAL STAGING

Staging in Pathology indicates timely progression of disease. This could be cancer staging (most famous) or other diseases staging (non-cancer)

IA. CANCER STAGING

IB. NON CANCER STAGING

IA. CANCER STAGING

*Tumour by simple definition is "**abnormal uncontrolled proliferation of cells**" with formation of a mass that is functionless and harmful!*
Note: In this book the word 'tumour' refers to **malignant tumour or cancer** (benign tumours are not staged or graded as a general concept)
*Staging in cancer is the **assessment of the degree of spread** of the tumour.*
Malignant tumours have the inherent ability to expand to nearby anatomical planes (direct spread) and/ or to involve remote anatomical structures/organs away from the original tumour (metastasis). Malignant cells can achieve this by the following:

1. The ability to **move**. Malignant tumour cells are motile with network of cytoplasmic filaments that can contract and relax, forming pseudopodia (feet-like structures).
2. The ability to **digest/degrade** the surrounding tissues through secretion of proteolytic enzymes including metalloproteinase, collagenase…etc.
3. The ability to synthesise and evoke the synthesis of its **own blood supply** by creating new blood vessels derived from surrounding innate blood vessels (angiogenesis)
4. The ability to **evade the immune system** and escape the destruction by immune cells. While travelling inside blood vessels they are veiled as platelets stick to their rough surfaces in the vascular lumen. Shedding of surfaces antigens and replacing them with new antigen is another way of hiding from immune cells.

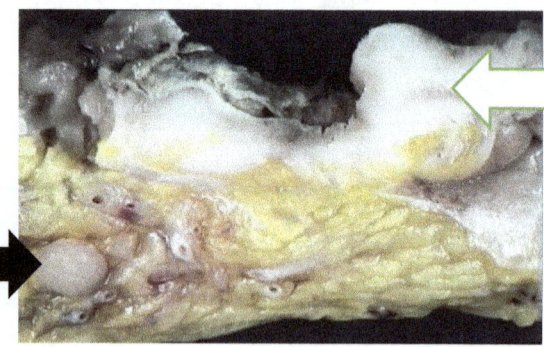

Colorectal cancer invading the muscularis propria (white filled arrow) and metastasize to lymph node (black arrow)

METHODS OF TUMOUR SPREAD

I. DIRECT TUMOUR SPREAD (T)/LOCAL INVASION

The tumour increases in size and invade the surrounding tissue ➜ reach lymphatic and blood vessels then metastasize to Lymph nodes and other organs. Tumour direct spread is an essential preliminary step before metastasis. The size of the tumour and the depth of invasion is directly proportionate to tumour ability to metastasise.

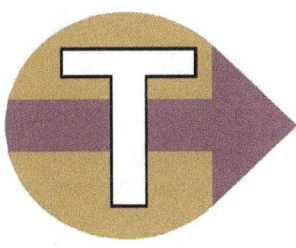

Steps of direct tumour spread:

- **Detachment:** the adhesion between tumour cells above basement membrane starts to disappear (loss of adhesion molecules, like E-cadherin), so cells can move individually.
- **Attachment:** cells then attach to the underlying basement membrane (BM) by new adhesion molecules adhere to laminin and collagen type IV of BM.
- **Penetration of BM:** tumour cells secrete enzymes (metalloproteinases, collagenase) to destroy the basement membrane (use laminin and collagen IV IHC or PAS stain to detect early invasion of BM).
- **Movement:** Tumour cells can move (motile) by pseudopodia, *a sign of malignancy* unlike normal cells. They move in the tissue helped by secretion of enzymes that destroys the tissues to reach lymphatic and blood vessels.

Effects of direct tumour spread:

Direct spread of the tumour corresponds clinically to the appearance of a destructive hard, painless mass (solid organs) or ulcer, perforation, obstruction or bleeding (hollow organs).

II.   METASTASIS (N, M):

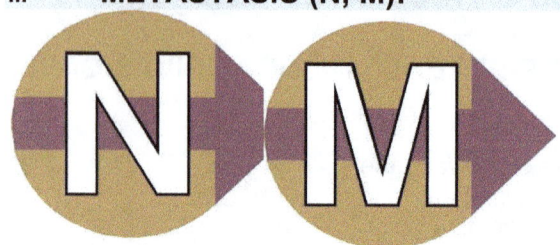

Metastasis = distant spread (there should be no direct continuity with the primary tumour). Metastasis (Greek = *displacement,* Plural: *metastases*), occasionally shortened as **mets.**

Note: direct spread from tumour to surrounding organs is not metastasis. Example: bowel cancer that penetrates directly to the liver or peritoneum is local invasion *NOT* metastasis. Another example is intramural tumour spread from cancer caecum to the ileum or appendix is direct invasion *NOT* metastasis.

Metastasis is the single most important difference between benign and malignant tumours.

The ability of the malignant tumours to metastasise varies from one tumour type to the other. On the other hand, some malignant tumours do not have capacity to metastasise and therefore recognised as "locally malignant tumours". Examples of the last category include gliomas, basal cell carcinoma, adamantinoma/ameloblastoma, giant cell tumours of bone craniopharyngeoma….etc.

When tumour cells metastasize, the new tumour is called a ***secondary, 2°, metastatic*** tumour ***implants, deposits***, or ***mets***, while the original tumour called ***primary tumour or 1°***

METHODS OF TUMOUR METASTASIS:

1.   LYMPHATIC SPREAD (N):

This is the preferred method of metastasis by **carcinoma**. However, some sarcomas may give lymph node deposits. Examples include synovial sarcoma and rhabdomyosarcoma.

Lymphatic spread of tumour can occur by any of the following methods:

• Tumour Emboli: solid masses of tumour cells migrating in lymphatic vessels and follow the lymphatic flow to regional LNs then from LNs to venous circulation➔ heart➔ other organs.

• Permeation: continuous cord of tumour cells where tumour cells proliferate while travelling inside the lymphatic vessels.

• Retrograde lymphatic spread: tumour emboli travel in the opposite direction to a common sharing tissue like skin, leading to ➔ skin nodules.

2. HAEMATOGENOUS (BLOOD) SPREAD (M):

This is the preferred method by **sarcoma**. However, some carcinomas are recognised by their propensity for haematogenous spread. Examples include follicular thyroid carcinoma, choriocarcinoma, hepatocellular carcinoma and renal cell carcinoma

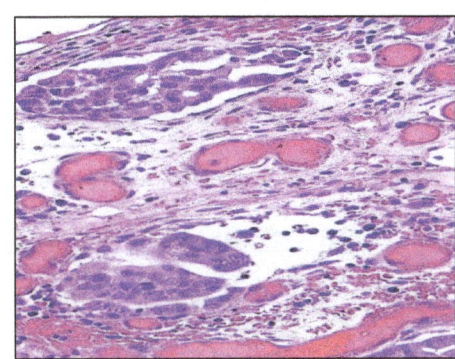

Multiple vascular tumour emboli

3. PERINEURAL SPREAD (Pn):

This is the preferred way of spread in prostatic adenocarcinoma and pancreatic adenocarcinoma

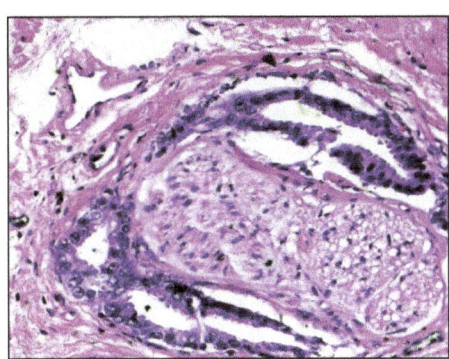

Perineural spared in prostatic adenocarcinoma

4. IMPLANTATION:

A tract of fine needle biopsy, or dislodged malignant cells during surgical operation could lead to tumour spread. Therefore it is essential to remove a cystic tumour (like ovarian) or bowel tumours with disrupting the tumour integrity. Surgical disruption of ovarian cancer will upstage the tumour from FIGO Ib to FIGO Ic due to possible tumour spread.

5. INOCULATION (CONTACT METASTASIS):

A tumour of one labia or lip transmitted to the normal facing side (kissing tumour)

6. TRANSLUMINAL SPREAD:

Tumour cells drop off from primary tumour in a hollow organ by gravity or through fluid (mucous, urine) or semi-solid material (stool) to come in contact with another part of the organ and form a secondary tumour (bronchus, Urinary system or intestine). This could explain synchronous multiple tumours. However, no clue to differentiate this from field effect, where multiple tumours could grow at the same time due to exposure of multiple tissue foci to the same mutagen.

7. TRANSCOELOMIC SPREAD:

Tumour cells separate from the original tumour in a cavity (pleural, peritoneal, dura..etc) and become lodged on the surface of another organ. Kruckenberg tumour of the ovary is an example, however there is a debate that Kruckenberg tumour may represent a lymphatic spread rather than real trans-coelomic spread.

EFFECTS OF TUMOUR ON THE BODY *(MECHANISMS OF MORBIDITY AND MORTALITY IN CANCER)*

I. EFFECT OF LOCAL/DIRECT TUMOUR SPREAD

A. SOLID ORGANS:

Examples:
Breast, liver, brain, spleen, kidney, ovary, prostate, bone or muscle.
Tumour appearance:
Non-capsulated, irregular outline, painless, hard, not well demarcated from surrounding + secondary changes (haemorrhage & necrosis)
Effects:
Disfiguring, asymmetry (especially breast)
Pressure effect:
Brain: increased intracranial pressure: headache, visual impairment, brain herniation➔ death
Lung: obstruction, collapse

B- HOLLOW ORGANS:

Examples:
Bowel, larynx, stomach, oesophagus, urinary bladder, uterus, ureters
Tumour Appearance:
1. Fungating / polypoid mass
2. Ulcer: Single, large, irregular outline with raised everted edge, necrotic and hard base
3. Diffuse infiltrating: Annular thickening of the wall

Effects:

- Lower GI (SI, colon): intestinal obstruction, Bleeding (bleeding per rectum, bright-fresh bleeding), perforation either at the tumour site or proximal due to obstruction
- Upper GI (stomach, oesophagus): Obstruction of the lumen➔ dysphagia, bleeding (hematemesis –digested brown blood)
- Uterus: abn bleeding, postmenopausal bleeding
- U bladder: haematuria, obstruction
- Larynx: hoarseness of voice, obstruction
- Organ perforation➔effusions in cavities like pleura or peritoneum
- Penetration to nearby organ➔causing adhesions and fistulae formation
- Invasion of large blood vessels➔ fatal bleeding, e.g., from lingual artery in cancer tongue or severe haemoptysis in lung cancer.

- Bilateral compression on both ureters by cervical carcinoma can →bilateral hydronephrosis and renal failure
- Invasion of nerves: neurological symptoms

II.   EFFECTS OF DISTANT SPREAD/TUMOUR METASTASIS

Metastasis is the most important negative prognostic factor in tumours
Tumours can harm the body through metastasis by the following:

- Failure of vital organs (liver, kidney , heart, brain)
- Pathological Fracture
- Enlarged lymph nodes (lymphadenopathy)
- Lungs: haemoptysis, cough and dyspnoea
- Liver: hepatomegaly (enlarged liver) and jaundice
- Bones: bone pain, fracture of affected bones
- Brain: signs of increased intracranial pressure (headaches, seizures, blindness)
- Effusions: pleura effusion, ascites
- Add to all of the above same effects of direct/local spread but in a remote location (away from primary tumour)

III.   PARA-NEOPLASTIC SYNDROME:

Definition: Signs and symptoms in cancer patients that cannot be explained by local spread or metastasis

- Acanthosis nigricans (grey-black skin patches): stomach, lung, uterus
- Anaemia: thymus
- Carcinoid syndrome
- Cushing's Syndrome: lung (small cell), pancreatic, neural,
- Dermatomyositis: lung, breast
- Hypercalcemia: due to destruction of bone by tumour or by secretion of PTH like substances by the tumour: SCC (lung, cervix, ovary), clear cell carcinoma (ovary, kidney), dysgerminoma
- Hypertrophic Osteoarthropathy (finger clubbing): lung
- Migratory Thrombophlebitis (Trousseau's): pancreas, lung
- Neuromyopathic syndromes (myasthenia gravis, cerebellar degeneration): lung, breast carcinoma, thymoma
- Polycythaemia: HCC, cerebellar haemangioma
- Syndrome of Inappropriate ADH: small cell carcinoma (lung), intracranial tumours

TNM STAGING OF TUMOURS (TNM 8th edition)

There are different systems of cancer spread assessment based on method and timing as follows

- cTNM: clinical examination/intra-operative or radiological
- pTNM: pathological staging (staging at excision, macroscopic and microscopic)
- ycTNM or ypTNM: post treatment/therapy (y) either clinical or pathological
- aTNM: staging at autopsy

Sites usually staged clinically include Cervix, Head and neck and Lymphomas.

Clinical staging used alone in the following cases:
- when no surgical treatment,
- adjuvant treatment done before surgery or
- deficient data to stage pathologically

The American Joint Committee on Cancer (AJCC) has established a TNM (tumour, node, and metastasis) classification system based on the same clinical and pathological staging information

TNM is the commonest and universal system used to in cancer staging.
For gynaecological tumours, there is in addition the FIGO classification
Duke's classification of colon cancer is no longer used.
No current TNM staging for adult brain tumours or phyllodes tumour of the breast.

Importance of have a universal TNM staging:

Tumour staging is the most important prognostic factor for any tumour. Therefore, the accuracy of staging procedure is crucial for determining the treatment options of the patient.

- Better Communication between medical practitioners
- Consistent nomenclature of cancer
- Agreed Staging & prognosis
- Treatment recommendations
- Efficiency of treatment

TNM is constantly changing due to variations in prognosis parameters after linking clinical data with pathological data.

The sourced if these information are:

TNM Data sources:

• NCDB (National Cancer Database). NCDB data are used to analyse and track patients with malignant neoplastic diseases, their treatments, and outcomes. Data represent more than 70 percent of newly diagnosed cancer cases nationwide and more than 34 million historical records.
• SEER (The Surveillance, Epidemiology, and End Results) program, which provides information on cancer statistics in USA.
• Multi-institutional databases
• International databases
• Publications

Discrepancy in tumour staging between pathologic, clinical and radiologic staging:

In some instances, there is difference between the tumour size evaluated clinically/radiologically and the pathologic macroscopic staging. The possible causes include:
- Time elapsed between the clinical/radiologic assessment and the sampling of the lesion for pathologic. The tumour size may increase before it is sampled specially in rapidly enlarging tumours.
- Measurement discrepancy: maximum dimension of the lesion is the most important and hence, the comparison should be done at this level or the three dimensions of the lesion should be mentioned
- Reaction of the surrounding tissue to the tumour, including fibrosis, necrosis, inflammation, haemorrhage and calcification may appear as part of the tumour.

In this book we will discuss the pathological cancer assessment (pTNM), NOT the clinical staging (unless there is no pathological staining is the organ/subject)

GENERAL RULES OF PATHOLOGICAL TNM CANCER STAGING:

LOCAL INVASION, PRIMARY TUMOUR STAGE) (T)

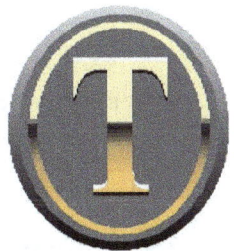

Assessment of local invasion (based on that the stage would be T1, T2, T3 or T4) depends on one or more of the following

1. Size of the tumour (maximum dimension or rarely in 3D as in cervix)
2. Extent of invasion measured digitally from a certain point (TT or DOI)
3. Extent of invasion defined anatomically (SM, MP, SS..etc)

TX Primary tumour cannot be evaluated
T0 No evidence of primary tumour
Tis Carcinoma in situ
Ta: malignant tumour that is exophytic like non-invasive papillary carcinoma and verrucous carcinoma
T(mi): microinvasive carcinoma, when the tumour extends to ≤1mm from the epithelial-stromal junction, e.g., in DCIS with microinvasion and cervical carcinoma

TUMOUR SIZE:

- **Maximum dimension** of all tumours is the main representative of the tumour except in cervical carcinoma where both transverse and longitudinal diameters are needed.

- **Size is crucial** in neuroendocrine tumours, renal cell carcinoma, cervical carcinoma, skin and head and neck tumours

- **Size of tumour does not matter** in hollow organ tumours in general including GI adenocarcinomas, urothelial carcinoma, uterine adenocarcinoma and ovarian tumours in addition to thymic carcinoma

TUMOUR EXTENT OF INVASION MEASURED DIGITALLY

1. Tumour thickness (TT):

In skin, TT measured from granular cell layer of adjacent normal epidermis to deepest point of the tumour

2. Depth of invasion (DOI):

DOI measured from Basement membrane of glands or surface epithelium. (epithelial–stromal junction) of nearby normal to deepest point of tumour. This is different from tumour thickness used in skin cancer which is measured from granular layer of adjacent normal skin.

EXTENT OF INVASION DEFINED ANATOMICALLY:

Most commonly used method.
Most of tumour local invasion depends on defining where the tumour extent is anatomically by crossing certain histological landmarks (examples in GI, submucosa, Muscularis propria..etc and in head and neck, cartilage, bones, major vessels or reaching deep anatomical planes like masseter muscle or brain.

MULTIPLE TUMOURS:

- Synchronous tumours of same type in one organ: classify by highest tumour stage, add (m) or (number of tumours) after tumour stage, e.g., T3 (m) or T2 (2)
- Synchronous bilateral tumours, classify individually, e.g. in both ovaries, both adrenals, both thyroid lobes or both liver lobes

PEARLS:

- No T1 in radical prostatectomy for adenocarcinoma
- No T1 or T2 in mucosal melanoma.
- No T3 or T4 for trophoblastic tumours.
- No T1 or T4 for primary peritoneal carcinoma.
- No T4 for ovarian or Fallopian tube tumours

- Multiple synchronous tumours of same type in one organ, stage using highest tumour stage and add **(m)** for multiple, e.g., T3 (m) or number of tumours , e.g., T3 (3)
- T4 generally indicates an advanced disease where:
  - T4a: Moderately advanced local disease = deep local invasion or visceral peritoneum, skin over the tumour

   o   T4b: Very advanced local disease = adjacent, vital organ or remote tissue invasion

DISCREPANCY BETWEEN MACROSCOPIC AND MICROSCOPIC TUMOUR SIZE:

Microscopic measurements are the most accurate, because it can precisely exclude the peri-tumoural tissues, including fibrosis and deduct it from the lesion size.

NODAL STAGE (N):

- pN0: no metastasis. However in breast, the presence of ITCs = pN0
- **N1-N3**: Involvement of regional LNs (size, side, number or anatomical site)
- Regional LNs differ according to anatomical site.

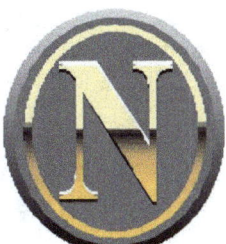

- Non regional LNs are considered distant metastasis (M) (for example in colorectal resection, peri-colic LNs are regional LNs, while coeliac LN is non regional).

Laterality in lymph nodes mets:

- Ipsi =same side
- Contra lateral = opposite side
- Midline nodes are considered ipsi nodes.

Size of pN: is the size of metastatic deposit is considered in staging, not of the size of the entire LN.
- **Micromets (mi):** met size is > 0.2 and < 2mm. size of met diagnosed after SLNB and lymphadenectomy (clinically occult)
- **Macromets:** clinical LN mets confirmed by bx or LN mets + extensive ENE (clinically apparent). Clinically detected = detected by imaging (not lymphoscintigraphy) or by clinical exam.
- **ENE** (extra-nodal extension) is an important parameter in nodal staging of Head and Neck carcinoma (new change in TNM8)
- Isolated tumour cells (ITC) = single tumour cells OR small clusters of cells < 0.2 mm in greatest OR < 200 cells in a single section.
- ITCs in Breast are = N0 while in Melanoma of the skin and Merkel Cell Carcinoma, ITC in a lymph node = N1.

- ITC in breast LN = pN0
- pN0 (i+) if ITC detected with IHC
- pN0 (mol+) if ITC detected by molecular study

Lymph node yield:
- The higher the number of dissected lymph nodes, the more accurate would be the assessment of nodal staging pathologically.
- Radical neck dissection specimen usually yields 10 or more LNs, while colectomy specimen yields a median of 12 LNs.
- Number of LNs is lower in post-neoadjuvant cancer resections.
- Following neo-adjuvant (chemo-radiotherapy), the lymph nodes shrink and are subject to fibrosis and calcification.
- Therefore multiple methods should be employed to increase the LN yield. These include:
  1. Longer fixation time with slicing of the fat
  2. Mixture of glacial acetic acid, buffered formalin and alcohol
  3. Xylene clearance method
  4. Embedding the entire fat especially fat around the vessels

MARGINS /COMPLETENESS OF RESECTION (R):

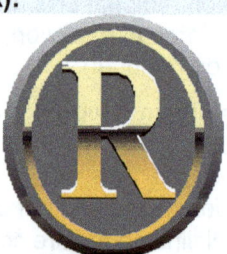

- Completeness of Resection **(R)**: this is required in many tumour resection staging and considered an important prognostic factor. This is divided into:
- **R0**: tumour completely excised locally
- **R1**: microscopic involvement of margin by tumour (to within 1mm)
- **R2**: macroscopic tumour left behind or gross involvement of margin

- Acceptable margin in head and neck tumours and melanomas is 5mm at least.
- In general a margin less than 1mm is considered to be an involved margin (R+) or high risk margin and further re-excision is recommended.
- Longitudinal margins are proximal and distal margins in tubular structures like small bowel, large bowel and ureter,
- R includes total circumferential/non peritonalised margin, e.g., total mesorectal excision **(TME) margin** in rectal cancer and total mesocolic resection **(TMC)** in other parts of the colon.
- Mesenteric fat margin is the non-peritonalised small bowel circumferential margin.

- Non peritonalised margins -need to be inked and assessed.
- Hepatic/liver non peritonalised margin need to be assessed in Gall bladder carcinoma.

POST TREATMENT STAGING (Y):

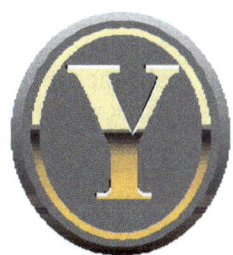

- New staging following radio-chemotherapy will be assigned "**y**". This could be pathological (yp) or clinical (yc) staging.
- Complete pathological response to chemoradiotherapy is labelled as **ypCR**.
- After radio/chemotherapy, new staging will be assigned **yTNM**. Retreatment staging, following recurrence will be assigned **rTNM**.

PERINEURAL INVASION (Pn):

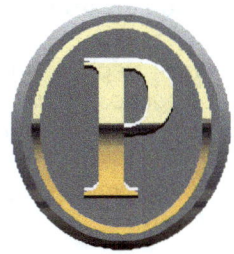

- Peri-neural Invasion "Pn", upgrades the staging in squamous cell carcinoma essential to be assessed in prostate and pancreas

METASTASIS (M):

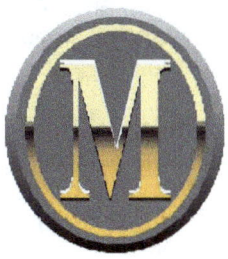

- No "MX" in TNM8.
- When M not mentioned in the text, M1= distant mets
- When N not mentioned in the text, N1= regional LNs mets

MICROSCOPIC FEATURES OF VALUE IN TUMOUR STAGING

Microscopic features are included in staging in certain tumours. Examples:
- Necrosis and grade in soft tissue, bone and penile tumours,

- Histological subtype: appendiceal carcinoid (well differentiated neuroendocrine tumour) staged differently from Goblet cell carcinoid
- Extra-nodal extension in LNs of head and neck.
- Depth of invasion (DOI) or tumour thickness (TT),
- ITCs and micromets,
- Tumour deposits (satellites) or in-transit mets in melanoma. Tumour satellites in CRC can change the nodal stage from pN1 to pN1c in absence of nodal metastasis
- Tumour histological type. Examples include staging of Merkel carcinoma of skin is different from poorly differentiated squamous cell carcinoma, both can only be differentiated microscopically.
- Histological/cytological evidence of metastasis can change the staging from pM0 to pM1

TNM GROUPING

Stage grouping:

Final stage = anatomical extent of disease, composed of T, N, and M categories in different combinations. Any M1= Stage IV. Stage grouping varies according to tumour type. In all TNM stage grouping, the final stage is IV, which indicates an advanced disease except in nephroblastoma "Wilms" and in case reports neuroblastoma, stage V assigned for a bilateral disease.

Prognostic Grouping:

• T, N, and M *plus* other prognostic factors, e.g., serum hormone level, mutations, patient's general condition, histologic grade and tumour type …etc.

Prognosis of a tumour can be scored BAD or GOOD based on many features including **morphologic** (e.g., tumour grading, tumour size), **clinical** (e.g., staging, recurrence, response to therapy, general condition of the patient), **investigations** (e.g., MRI showing tumour spread, high level of tumour markers), **immunohistochemistry** (e.g., HER2, ER or Ki-67 status in breast cancer) or **molecular** assay (e.g., N-Myc amplification in neuroblastoma, BRCA1 mutation in breast cancer). The following classification of prognostic factors is applicable to most of the tumours. Differences between tumours regarding prognostic factors are just in the subtitles

SUMMARY OF PATHOLOGICAL TNM, 8TH EDITION

HEAD AND NECK TUMOURS

- Head & neck carcinomas only included in the following section. Other tumours like lymphoma or soft issue tumours are staged differently.
- T size not considered in mucosal melanoma, nasal sinuses, nasopharynx and larynx carcinomas.
- Prognostic factors include: histologic tumour grade, LVI, size of LN metastatic deposit, extra-nodal extension (ENE), and resection margins status (5mm is safe clear margin).
- Carotid involvement is by encasing not by invading carotid artery

The anatomical sites of H&N are:
- Lip and oral cavity
- Pharynx: oropharynx (p16 negative and p16 positive), nasopharynx, hypopharynx
- Larynx: supraglottis, glottis, subglottis
- Nasal cavity and paranasal sinuses (maxillary and ethmoid sinus)
- Unknown primary carcinoma – cervical nodes
- Malignant melanoma of upper aerodigestive tract
- Major salivary glands
- Thyroid gland

LIP, ORAL CAVITY

T1: ≤2cm + DOI ≤5mm
T2: ≤2cm + DOI > 5-10mm or > 2 - 4 cm + DOI <10mm
T3: > 4cm or DOI >10mm
T4 differs according to the anatomical site:
- **T4a (lip):** skin of nose/chin, inferior alveolar nerve, mouth floor or through cortical bone
- **T4a (oral cavity):** skin of face, deep tongue muscles, maxillary sinus or through cortical bone.
- **T4b (lip+oral):** masticular space, pterygoid plates, skull base or carotid.

Notes:
Oral cavity involves the tongue, floor of the mouth
Superficial bone erosion ≠T4

Lip has three compartments, each staged differently:
-Vermilion surface and commissures, staged under the *lip* as above
-Hair bearing area of the lip is staged under *skin cancer*
-Inner mucosal surface of the lip, staged under *oral cavity*

PHARYNX

Oropharynx (oropharyngeal carcinoma, OPC)

Classified based on p16 positivity (HPV status) into

HPV+ OPC (*Oropharynx – p16- Positive Tumours*)
T stage
T1: ≤2cm
T2: > 2 - 4 cm
T3: > 4cm OR extension to lingual surface of epiglottis (mucosa)
T4: T invades larynx, deep muscle of tongue, pterygoid plates or muscles, hard-palate, mandible, nasopharynx, skull base or encases carotid artery
N stage:
Like nodal staging for all H&N (ENE does not change the stage)

HPV- OPC (*Oropharynx – p16- Negative Tumours*)
T stage
T1, T2 and T3 staged as HPV+ OPC
- **T4a** : larynx, medial pterygoid, deep tongue muscles, hard palate or mandible
- **T4b**: lateral pterygoid, skull base, nasopharynx or carotid (encasement)

Hypopharynx

T1: ≤2cm OR 1 subsite
T2: > 2 - 4 cm OR > 1 subsite
T3: > 4cm OR fixation of hemilarynx OR extension to oesophagus
T4a: cricoid, hyoid, thyroid cartilage, or central soft tissue
T4b: pre-vertebral fascia, carotid, or mediastinum

Nasopharynx

T1: Nasopharynx, oropharynx or nasal Cavity. No para-pharyngeal extension
T2: Para-pharyngeal extension OR pterygoid muscles (lat/med)
T3: invasion of bones of skull base, pterygoid or paranasal sinuses

T4: intracranial, cranial nerves, hypopharynx, parotid or beyond lat. Surface of lat. pterygoid muscle

NASAL CAVITY AND PARANASAL SINUSES

Nasal Cavity and Ethmoid Sinus
T1: 1 subsite
T2: 2 subsites
T3: orbit, maxillary sinus, palate, cribriform plate
Maxillary Sinus
T1: Mucosa
T2: Bones (inferior or medial wall, hard palate, middle nasal meatus)
T3: Posterior wall sinus, orbit (inferior /medial wall), subcutaneous
For All Nasal Cavity and paranasal sinuses
T4a: Anterior orbit, anterior cranial fossa or skin
T4b: Superior orbit, middle cranial fossa, brain

CARCINOMA OF UNKNOWN PRIMARY (CUP)

If LN mets are squamous carcinoma positive for HPV (p16+): stage nodal stage as for HPV+ OPC (90% of CUP are HPV+ OPC). If EBV positive, stage nodal stage as nasopharyngeal carcinoma. Both are called viral-mediated unknown primary and will be assigned T0.
If HPV and EBV are negative (TX) the tumour will be from other subsites. Refer to below nodal stage for both HPV+OPC and Nasopharyngeal carcinoma

MUCOSAL MELANOMA OF AERODIGESTIVE TRACT

No T1 or T2 in mucosal melanoma staging, due to their aggressiveness
T3: Epithelium/ submucosa
T4a: Deep local invasion (soft tissue, cartilage, bone) or overlying skin
T4b: _Adjacent_ (skull base, carotid, masticator or pre-vertebral space), _vital_ (skull contents: brain, dura or lower cranial nerves 9, 10, 11, 12) or _remote structures_ (mediastinum)

LARYNX

Supraglottis
T1: 1 subsite, N mobility
T2: >1subsite, N mobility
T3: Cord fixation or deep invasion (post-cricoid, pre-epiglottic, thyroid)
Glottis

T1: vocal cord (s), N mobility
T1a: 1 cord
T1b: both cords
T2: Supra/ subglottis, impaired mobility
T3: cord fixation, para-glottic space, thyroid cartilage
Subglottis
T1: subglottis,
T2: vocal cord(s) + N/ impaired mobility
T3: Cord fixation
For All Larynx
T4a: deep local (Soft tissues, tongue, strap muscles, thyroid, oesophagus)
T4b: adjacent (Pre-vertebral space), vital (carotid), remote (mediastinum)

SALIVARY GLANDS

T1: ≤ 2 cm
T2: >2 - 4 cm
T3: >4 OR any size + extra-parenchymal extension
T4a: Deep local invasion (mandible, ear, facial nerve) or overlying skin
T4b: Adjacent (skull, pterygoid plates) or vital (carotid)
Note: extraparenchymal extension (T3) evaluated clinically or macroscopic NOT microscopic.

THYROID

All subtypes: Papillary/follicular (include Hurthle)/medullary/Anaplastic

T1: ≤ 2cm, intra-thyroid
T1a: ≤ 1cm, intra-thyroid
T1b: >1-2cm, intra-thyroid
T2: >2-4cm, intra-thyroid
T3a: >4 cm limited to the thyroid
T3b: any size + gross extra-thyroidal extension invading only strap muscles
T4a: invades larynx, trachea, oesophagus, recurrent laryngeal nerve or subcutaneous
T4b: invades pre-vertebral fascia, mediastinal vessels or encases carotid

Prognostic factors

Papillary and Follicular: extra thyroid extension, age >55 (poor), margin involvement
Medullary Cancer: Pre and postoperative calcitonin and CEA, Age, and margin

Regional Lymph Nodes of Head and Neck

- Cervical LN dissection includes levels I-VII:

Level 1 (I): submental & submandibular
Level 2 (II): Upper jugular
Level 3 (III): Mid-jugular
Level 4 (IV): Lower jugular
Level 5 (V): Posterior triangle LNs
Level 6 (VI): Pre-laryngeal, Pre-tracheal & Para-tracheal
Level 7 (VII): Upper mediastinal

- Selective neck dissection ≥10 LNs.
- Radical or modified radical neck dissection specimen ≥15 LNs

Lip, oral cavity, Hypopharynx and HPV+ OPC, salivary gland and Larynx

N1: Ipsi single ≤3 cm (ENE-)
N2a: Ipsi single, ≤3 cm (ENE+) or >3 - 6 cm (ENE-)
N2b: Ipsi multiple, any ≤6 cm (ENE-)
N2c: Bilateral or contra, any ≤6 cm (ENE-)
N3a: any >6 cm (ENE-)
pN3b: >3 cm (ENE+) or, multiple ipsi, or any contra or bilateral node(s) (ENE+)

HPV- OPC

N1:1 - 4 LN
N2: ≥ 5 LNs

Nasopharynx
N1: Unilat. cervical, unilat./bilat. Retro-pharyngeal ≤ 6 cm above cricoid cartilage (caudal end)
N2: Bilat. cervical ≤ 6 cm above cricoid cartilage (caudal end)
N3: cervical LN (s)>6 cm or extension below cricoid cartilage (caudal end)
Mucosal Melanoma:
N1: regional LN (s)

Thyroid:
N1a: cervical level VI (pre/para-tracheal, pre-laryngeal) or superior mediastinum
N1b: cervical other levels I, II, III, IV or V (uni-, bi-, or contra), or retropharyngeal

GASTROINTESTINAL TRACT

Oesophageal vs. gastric

Stage as oesophageal if:
- T epicentre within 2 cm of GOJ and extends into oesophagus
- T involving GOJ with epicentre in proximal 2 cm of cardia (Siewert types I/II)

Stage as gastric if T epicentre > 2 cm distal to GOJ even if GOJ involved.

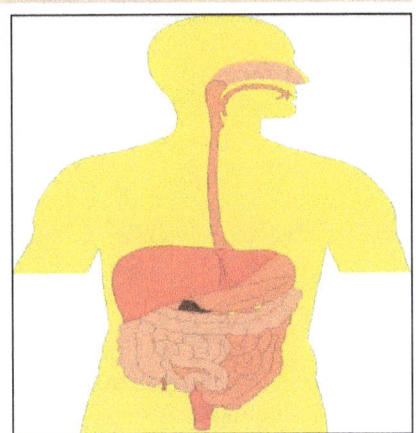

Oesophagus

Applies for adenoca and SCC

Tis: High-grade dysplasia/ CIS
T1: LP or SM (**T1a:** LP/MM, **T1b**: SM)
T2: MP
T3: Adventitia
T4: Adjacent
T4a: Pleura, pericardium, diaphragm
T4b: other; aorta, vertebral body, trachea
N1: 1-2 LN
N2: 3-6 LN
N3: ≥ 7 LN
Prognostic factors: Her2 (adenoca) LVI, margins, CEA

Stomach

Tis: CIS/ high grade dysplasia
T1: LP or SM (T1a: LP, **T1b**: SM)
T2: MP
T3: SS (also extension to lesser /greater omentum without perforation)
T4a: perforates serosa
T4b: invades adjacent structures
N1: 1 - 2 LNs, **N2**: 3 -6 LNs, **N3a:** 7 - 15 LNs, **N3b**: ≥ 16 LNs
M1: distant mets, positive peritoneal cytology or peritoneal bx

Prognostic factors: Her2, age, site in the stomach, margins, Asian vs non-Asian

Note: 16 or more LNs is ideal in the specimen

Small Intestine

Non-ampullary duodenum, Jejunum and ileum

Tis: CIS
T1: LP/SM
T2: MP
T3: SS, non-peritonealised peri-muscular tissues (mesentery, retroperitoneum) ≤2 cm
T4: Visceral peritoneum, adjacent structures (incl. mesentery, retroperitoneum) >2 cm
N1:1-2LNs
N2: ≥3LNs

Number of LNs expected in the specimen 6 or more

Ampulla of Vater (AOV)

T1a: limited to ampulla /sphincter of Oddi
T1b: to duodenal SM
T2: to duodenal MP
T3: pancreas
T3a: pancreas to ≤5mm
T3b: pancreas >5mm OR peripancreatic tissue OR duodenal serosa
T4: SMA OR coeliac axis OR common hepatic a
N1: 1-2 LNs
N2: ≥ 3 LNs

Pancreas

Pancreatic adenocarcinoma (exocrine). Neuroendocrine tumours staged in NET.

Tis: CIS (high grade PanIN- PanIN III)
T1 :≤2 cm
T1a:≤ 0.5 cm
T1b: 0.5 - 1 cm

T1c >1-2 cm
T2: > 2 - 4 cm
T3: > 4 cm
T4: coeliac axis, SMA and/or common hepatic artery
N1:1- 3 LNs
N2: >4LNs

Prognostic factors: Preoperative CA 19-9 & CEA

Ideal LNs in the specimen 12 LNs or more

Colon-Rectum

T1: SM
T2: MP
T3: SS, non-peritonealised peri-colic/peri-rectal tissues
T4a: perforates visceral peritoneum
T4b: invades other organs
N1: 1 -3 LNs (**N1a**: 1 LN, **N1b**: 2 – 3 LNs, **N1c:** Satellites in SS, without LN mets)
N2: ≥ 4 LNs (N2a: 4 – 6 LNs, **N2b**:≥ 7 LNs)
M1: Distant mets:
M1a: 1 organ or non-regional LNs (not peritoneum)
M1b: > 1 organ (not peritoneum)
M1c: peritoneal mets

Note: **Tumour deposits** (satellites): irregular nodules in subserosal fat not continuous with main tumour. *By exclusion, they are not LN or EMVI (venous invasion), LVI (small tumour emboli) or perineural invasion.* Presence of satellites in absence of LN mets = N1c

Prognostic factors include: LVI, perineural Invasion, grade, tumour budding, perforation, KRAS, MSI, BRAF, age and race.

Note: extraction of 12 or more LNs is ideal in colorectum specimen

Appendix

Adenocarcinoma (non-mucinous and mucinous including goblet cell carcinoid):
T1: SM
T2: MP
T3: SS, or meso-appendix

T4a: Perforates visceral peritoneum (for mucinous tumours, peritoneal spread within right lower quadrant "RLQ")
T4b: other adjacent organs
N1: 1- 3 LN, **N2:** > 3 LN
M1a: Intra-peritoneal mets beyond RLQ
M1b: Non-peritoneal mets

Notes:
Well differentiated NET is staged under NET.
Low-grade appendiceal mucinous neoplasm confined to the appendix up to MP **(LAMN) is Tis**.
LAMN invading SS = T3 or serosa = T4a.

For LAMN, M1: Distant metastasis
       M1a: acellular mucin in the peritoneum
       M1b: mucinous epithelium in the peritoneum
       M1c: mets to other organs

Anal canal

Definition: Tumours within 5 cm from anal margin
Tis: CIS (Bowen's, HSIL, AIN II-III)
T1: ≤2cm
T2: >2-5 cm
T3: >5 cm
T4: Adjacent organ (s)
N1a: inguinal, meso-rectal and OR internal iliac
N1b: external iliac
N1c: external iliac AND inguinal, mesorectal AND OR internal iliac

Prognostic factors : Skin ulceration, Sphincter invasion, T size >5 cm, immunodeficiency, Long term corticosteroids, HIV, SCC antigen (SCC Ag), presence of herpes simplex virus (HSV), anaemia

Gastrointestinal Stomal Tumour (GIST)

T1: ≤ 2 cm,
T2: > 2 – 5 cm,
T3: > 5 – 10 cm,
T4: > 10 cm

Grading:
- **Low grade**: mitosis ≤5/50hpf
- **High grade**: mitosis >5/50hpf. HPF= 40x (5mm^2)

Stage grouping includes mitotic rate and differs in according to site

- Stage grouping includes mitotic rate and differs in according to site (stomach more benign than intestine)
- Use of CD117 and DOG-1 is essential
- CD117 negative GIST exists, but > 50% of them are DOG-1 (+). Double negative GIST is 2% are present and diagnosed based on morphology.
- Treatment by tyrosine kinase inhibitors, e.g., Imatinib
- Types : spindle, epithelioid or mixed

Prognostic factors: Histological type, Size of tumour, Depth of invasion, Grade (well to poorly differentiated), Mitotic rate, Presence of *c Kit* mutation or *PDGFRA* gene

NEUROENDOCRINE TUMOURS OF GIT

WELL- DIFFERENTIATED NET (G1 and G2) OF GIT AND PANCREAS:

NET = Neuroendocrine tumours
- Staging here applies only to Well diff NET = carcinoid (G1) +atypical carcinoid (G2) of GIT and Pancreas
- **Small cell or large cell NEC (Grade 3) of any site**: staged as carcinoma
- Mucinous (goblet) carcinoid, NOW CALLED GOBLET CELL ADENOCARCINOMA staged as appendiceal carcinoma
- **Lung** NET: staged as lung carcinoma
- **Skin:** Merkel cell carcinoma has a separate staging under skin tumours

GRADING OF NET based on the Ki-67 index. Ki-67 index = % of Ki-67 (+) cells/2000 cells. Grade 1= <3%, Grade 2= 3-20%, Grade 3= >20%
- 10 HPF (high power fields) = 2 X mm^2; at least 40 fields (at 40× magnification) evaluated in areas of highest mitotic density.
- MIB1 antibody; % of 500–2000 tumour cells in areas of highest nuclear labelling.

APPENDIX NET
T1: ≤ 2 cm
T2: > 2 – 4 cm OR minimal invasions of subserosa < 3 mm
T3: > 4 cm or invasion of mesoappendix (subserosal)
T4: Perforates serosa or other organs **Not** by direct mural extension)

STOMACH NET
T1: LP/SM & ≤ 1 cm,
T2: MP or > 1 cm
T3: SS,
T4: Perforates serosa or other organs

DUODENAL/AMPULLARY NET
T1: Duodenal: LP/SM & ≤ 1 cm,
T2: Duodenal: MP or > 1 cm

T1: Ampullary: confined within sphincter of Oddi & ≤ 1 cm,
T2: Ampullary: invades through sphincter into duodenal SM or MP OR >1cm
T3: both: pancreas or peripancreatic adipose tissue
T4: both: serosa or invades other organs

JEJUNUM/ILEUM NET

T1: LP/SM & ≤ 1 cm
T2: MP or > 1 cm
T3: SS
T4: serosa or other organs

PANCREAS NET

T1: limited to pancreas & ≤2 cm
T2: limited to pancreas & > 2cm- 4 cm
T3: limited to pancreas & >4 or invading duodenum or bile duct (Invasion of peripancreatic fat is T3)
T4: serosa or other organs
Pancreatic NET prognostic factors: Endocrine: Preoperative plasma chromogranin A level + Mitotic count

COLON/RECTUM NET

T1: LP/SM & ≤2cm (**T1a:** < 1 cm, **T1b**: 1 - 2 cm)
T2: MP or > 2 cm
T3: SS
T4: serosa or other organs

Nodal and distant metastasis staging of all NET of GI and pancreas are similar as follows (except Jejunum and Ileum N stage):

N1: Regional lymph node metastasis
M1a: Hepatic mets
M1b: Extrahepatic mets
M1c: Hepatic + extrahepatic mets
Jejunum and Ileum NET Nodal stage:
N1: <12 LNs without mesenteric mass > 2 cm
N2: ≥12 LNs and/or mesenteric mass > 2 cm

LIVER, BILE DUCTS & GALL BLADDER

Hepatocellular Carcinoma (HCC)

T1a: single ≤ 2 cm ± LVI
T1b: single > 2cm, no LVI
T2: single > 2cm + LVI *OR* multiple, any < 5 cm,
T3: multiple, any >5 cm
T4: invades major branch of portal v OR hepatic vein + adjacent organ (not GB) OR visceral peritoneum invasion
N1: regional LN mets
Note: 3 or more LNs is ideal in the specimen

Prognostic factors: Vascular invasion, Size >5 cm, multiplicity, liver fibrosis, high Ki67 index, abnormal liver function, portal hypertension, residual tumour after treatment, high AFP level, neutrophil to lymphocyte ratio

Intrahepatic cholangiocarcinoma

T1a: single ≤ 5 cm, no LVI
T1b: single > 5 cm, no LVI
T2: single + LVI or multiple tumours, ± LVI
T3: Tumour perforating the visceral peritoneum
T4: Tumour involving local extrahepatic structures by direct hepatic invasion
N1: regional LN mets

Note: 6 or more LNs is ideal in the specimen

Peri-hilar = Proximal Extrahepatic bile ducts (hilar) (including Rt, Lt and common hepatic ducts)

T1: ductal wall
T2a: beyond ductal wall to fat
T2b: to surrounding liver
T3: unilat portal v/hepatic a branches,
T4: main portal vein, bilat branches /large bile radicals

N1: 1–3 LNs
N2: ≥ 4 LNs
Note: 15 or more LNs is ideal in the specimen

Distal Extrahepatic bile ducts, (from cystic duct insertion to common hepatic duct)

T1: Ductal wall to depth <5mm
T2: Beyond ductal wall to depth 5-12mm
T3: Beyond ductal wall to depth >12mm
T4: Celiac axis, or SMA (sup. mesenteric artery), common hepatic a
N1: 1–3 LNs
N2: ≥ 4 LNs

Note: 12 or more LNs is ideal in the specimen

Gall bladder carcinoma:

Tis: CIS,
T1a: LP, **T1b:** MP,
T2: invades perimuscular CT,
       T2a: perimuscular CT on peritoneal side
       T2b perimuscular CT on hepatic side
T3: perforates serosa OR to liver OR 1 adjacent organ
T4: portal v, hepatic a, or ≥2 adjacent organs

N1: 1–3 LNs
N2: ≥ 4 LNs
Note: 6 or more LNs is ideal in the specimen

RESPIRATORY TRACT (lower)

Lung, NSCC, SCC and carcinoid

Staging includes Non small cell carcinoma (NSCC, adenocarcinoma and Squamous), Small cell carcinoma (SCC) and Carcinoid

Tis: adca in situ and SCC in situ
T1: ≤3 cm - not in main bronchus
    T1mi: minimally invasive adenoca
    T1b: >1cm - 2 cm
    T1c: >2cm - 3cm
T2: >3cm - 5cm OR T in main bronchus but away from carina OR invades visceral pleura OR partial atelectasis
    T2a: >3 - 4 cm
    T2b: >4 -5 cm
T3: >5- 7 cm OR T invades parietal pleura, chest wall, phrenic n, Parietal pericardium, OR separate nodule(s) in same lobe
T4: >7cm OR T invades: diaphragm, mediastinum (heart, carina, great vessels, trachea recurrent n, oesophagus) OR separate nodules in different ipsi lobe
N1: Ipsi peribronchial/ hilar LN
N2: Ipsi mediastinal/ subcarinal LN
N3: Contra mediastinal, hilar, scalene or supraclav LN.
Regional lymph nodes
N1 nodes: 10= Hilar, 11= Inter-lobar (peri-bronchial), Intrapulmonary including 12= Lobar, 13= Segmental, 14= Subsegmental)
N2 nodes: 1= Highest mediastinal, 2 =Upper paratracheal, 3 =Pre-vascular and retro-tracheal, 4 =Lower para-tracheal, 5= Subaortic, 6= Para-aortic, 7= Subcarinal, 8= Para-oesophageal, 9= Pulmonary ligament
N3 nodes: any **contra** LNs

M1a: tumour nodule(s) in contra. Lung lobe, pleural/pericardial nodules or malignant pleural/pericardial effusion
M1b: 1 extrathoracic met in 1 organ
M1c: Multiple extrathoracic metastasis in a single or multiple organs

Pleural mesothelioma

T1: ipsi. pleura (parietal or visceral) (no visceral or mediastinal diaphragmatic pleura)
T2: lung or diaphragm
T3: endothoracic fascia OR mediastinal fat OR focal chest wall soft tissue OR non-transmural pericardium (advanced but resectable)
T4: Contra pleura OR chest wall OR peritoneum OR mediastinum, myocardium OR spine OR malignant pericardial effusion (advanced & non-resectable)
N1: Ipsi intrathoracic (bronchopulmonary, hilar, ... etc)
N2: contra intrathoracic OR Supraclav- ipsi/contra.

Thymic Tumours

Staging applies to thymomas, thymic carcinomas and NET of the thymus.

T1: Tumour encapsulated or extending into the mediastinal fat
T1a: No mediastinal pleural involvement
T1b: Invasion of mediastinal pleura
T2: pericardium (partial or full thickness).
T3: lung OR brachiocephalic vein, OR superior vena cava OR phrenic nerve, OR chest wall OR pulmonary artery/vein (extra-pericardial).
T4: Aorta OR arch vessels OR pulmonary artery (intra-pericardial) OR myocardium OR trachea, OR oesophagus
N1: anterior (peri-thymic)
N2: deep intrathoracic or cervical
M1a: Separate pleural or pericardial nodule(s)
M1b: mets beyond pleura or pericardium

FEMALE ORGANS

A-BREAST

Tis (DCIS / LCIS/Paget's)
T1: tumour in mm (**T1mi**:≤ 1mm, **T1a**: >1- 5mm, **T1b**: >5 -10mm, **T1c**: >10 -20mm)
T2: > 2-5cm,
T3: > 5cm
T4a: Chest wall (bone and cartilage NOT pectoralis muscle),
T4b: Skin (ulcer, nodules or oedema "peau d'orange". Note: Dermis invasion only ≠ T4. The epidermis should be ulcerated to consider T4b),
T4c: T4a + T4b,
T4d: Inflammatory carcinoma (clinically= erythema + oedema "peau d'orange" ≥1/3 breast skin, pathologically dermal lymphatic emboli + invasive tumour)
N1mi: micromets = >0.2 or >200cells, but any <2mm.
ITCs (isolated tumour cells) : < 0.2 mm or < 200 cells in one section (considered N0, or N0 (i+) if detected only by IHC). ITCs are not included in the staging **(Compare with melanoma staging) but counted as positive lymph node (e.g., 1/19 LN but N0)**

N1a: 1-3 axillary, >2mm (macromets)
N1b: internal mammary mets by SLNB, not clinically
N1c: 1-3 axillary + internal mammary mets by SLNB, occult clinically
N2a: 4-9 axillary
N2b: Internal mammary, clinically
N3a: ≥10 axillary, or infraclav
N3b: internal mammary, clinically or >3 axillary + internal mammary, by SLNB, occult clinically
N3c: supraclav

Breast regional LNs (all ipsi):
1. **Axillary** (Note: intra-mammary LN is counted as an axillary LN):
Level1 (low axilla)
Level2 (mid axilla) include Rotter [interpectoral LN]
Level3 (apical axilla), include infraclav
2. **Internal mammary** LNs (rarely sampled)
3. **Supraclav** LN
Any other LNs, including cervical or contra LNs = **M1** (this is problematic in bilateral breast cancer)

Definitions:

N1& N2: Level1& 2 axillary,
N3: Level3, infraclav, supraclav, internal mammary.
cM0(i+): Molecularly/micro-detected tumour cells in circulating blood, bone marrow or other non-regional nodal tissue < 0.2 mm in patient without symptoms or signs of metastases
M1: mets detected clinically/ radiographic or histologically > 0.2 mm

PEARLS
MICROINVASION (Tmi) = tumour invasion of ≤ 1mm (0.1cm) from basement membrane of the duct.
If multiple Tmi, the largest tumour is considered. Multiplicity should be mentioned in the report

ypN: Post- treatment Nodal staging
N (sn): when staging based only on sentinel LN

NOTTINGHAM PROGNOSTIC INDEX (NPI) = (0.2 x tumour diameter in cms) + lymph node stage + tumour grade

- **Lymph node stage:** (1 = no nodes affected, 2 = up to 3 nodes affected, 3 = more than 3 nodes affected
- **Tumour grade:** (1 = for grade I or less, 2 = for grade II, 3 = for grade III)

PROGNOSTIC FACTORS:
ER/ HER2 status, grade, LVI, margin status, age, pre or post-menopausal, Hx of radiation, *BRCA1* or *2* mutation, obesity, hormone replacement therapy, Ki 67 index

B- FEMALE GENITAL TRACT

- Staging is predominantly clinical
- FIGO staging also included in Latin numbers
- No FIGO 0
- **Depth of invasion (DOI)** measured from Basement membrane of glands or surface epith. (epithelial–stromal junction) of nearby normal to deepest point of tumour. This is different from tumour thickness used in skin cancer which is measured from granular layer of N skin.

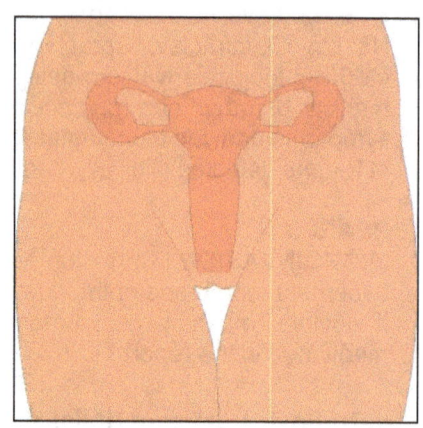

Vulva

Tis: CIS (VIN3)
T1: Confined to vulva/perineum
T1a: DOI < 2 cm + invasion < 1.0 mm (IA), **T1b: DOI** > 2 cm or invasion > 1.0 mm (IB)
T2: Lower urethra/vagina/anus (II)
T3: Upper urethra/vagina, bladder, rectal/mucosa, bone, fixed to pelvic bone (IVA)
N1a: 1-2 LNs, any < 5 mm
N1b: 1LN ≥ 5 mm
N2a: ≥3 LNs any < 5 mm
N2b: ≥2 LNs ≥ 5 mm
N2c: ENE (extra-nodal extension)
N3: Fixed, ulcerated

Vagina

Tis: CIS (VAIN3)
T1: Vaginal wall (FIGO I),
T2: Paravaginal tissue (FIGO II),
T3: pelvic wall (FIGO III),
T4: Mucosa of bladder/rectum, beyond pelvis (FIGO IVA)

Cervix

T1: Confined to uterus
T1a: microscopic only (clinically occult)
    T1a1: DOI <3 mm, horizontal <7 mm
    T1a2: DOI >3-5 mm, horizontal <7mm
T1b: DOI > T1a2, or clinically detected
    T1b1 <4cm
    T1b2: >4 cm
T2: Beyond uterus but not pelvic wall or lower 1/3 vagina
    T2a: No parametrium
    T2b: Parametrium
T3: Lower 1/3 vagina/pelvic wall/hydronephrosis
    T3a: Lower 1/3 vagina
    T3b: Pelvic wall/hydronephrosis
T4: Mucosa of bladder/rectum; beyond true pelvis

Note: FIGO follows TNM exactly, e.g., T1b2 = IB2, except T4=IVA
IVB= M1

LVI or uterine body-corpus involvement do not affect stage

Prognostic Factors:
Poor: bilateral disease, Parametrial invasion, LVI, positive margins, HIV, obesity, Anaemia, persistence of HPV
Other: VEGF, serum MyoDI,

UTERINE BODY-CORPUS

Adenocarcinoma and carcinosarcoma (MMMT)

T1: within corpus
T1a: endometrium or < ½ myometrium
T1b: ≥ ½ myometrium
T2: cervical stroma (glandular invasion only = T1)
T3: Local or regional
T3a: serosa or adnexa
T3b: vagina or parametrium
T4: mucosa of bladder/rectum
N1: pelvic LNs
N2: para-aortic LNs
M1: Inguinal LNs, peritoneum or distant organs e.g., lung, liver

Leiomyosarcoma and Endometrial stromal sarcoma

T1: uterus only
T1a: ≤ 5 cm
T1b: > 5 cm
T2: beyond uterus, in pelvis
T2a: Adnexa,
T2b: Other pelvic tissues
T3: abdominal tissues
T3a: 1 site
T3b: > 1 site
T4: bladder or rectum

Adenosarcoma

T1: within corpus
T1a: endometrium or
T1b :< ½ myometrium
T1c: ≥ ½ myometrium
T2: beyond uterus, in pelvis
T2a: Adnexa,
T2b: Other pelvic tissues
T3: abdominal tissues
T3a: 1 site
T3b: > 1 site
T4: bladder/rectum
N1: pelvic LNs
Note: FIGO staging like cervix

Gestational Trophoblastic Tumours

T1: Confined to uterus
T2: Other genital structures
M1a: Mets to lung(s)
M1b: Other distant mets
Stage grouping includes prognostic score index; **Low risk:** ≤ 6, **High risk:** ≥ 7
Prognostic score involves age, site/no. of mets. Pre-Tx hCG level, size of T, previous failed chemo, interval to pregnancy

OVARY, FALLOPIAN TUBES AND PRIMARY (1°) PERITONEAL

Classification involves:
- Mg ovarian Ts (epithelial and stromal) + borderline + low mg potential
- Fallopian tubes and peritoneum (Müllerian origin)

T1 (FIGO I): Limited to ovary (1 or both) or FT (1 or both)

    T1a: 1 ovary, capsule intact or 1 FT surface (neg perit wash)

    T1b: 2 ovaries, capsule intact or 2 FT surface (neg perit wash)

    T1c: Same as T1b with one of the following:

        T1c1: Surgical spill

        T1c2: Capsule ruptured before surgery

        T1c3: positive peritoneal wash

T2 (FIGO II): Pelvic extension (below pelvic brim) OR **1° peritoneal cancer**

    T2a: Uterus, FT(s) OR ovary (s)

    T2b: Other pelvic organs

T3 (FIGO III): Peritoneal mets, extrapelvic (H&E or mg cytology) or retroperitoneal LNs

    T3a: microscopic extrapelvic peritoneal mets +/- retroperitoneal LN, or bowel

    T3b: Macroscopic extrapelvic peritoneal mets ≤ 2 cm, +/- retroperitoneal LN, or bowel

    T3c: like T3b, >2cm (include capsular not parenchymal mets of liver OR spleen)

N1: Retroperitoneal LN mets only (also = T3)

    N1a: ≤ 10 mm

    N1b: >10 mm

M1: Distant mets (excludes peritoneal mets= T3)

    M1a: mg pleural cytology

    M1b: parenchymal mets to liver or spleen or extra abdominal organs OR non regional LNs: e.g., inguinal LNs or extra-abdominal LNs

Prognostic Factors: Histological type, Grade, DNA ploidy, CA125, *BRCA1* mutation, Tumour angiogenesis markers, p53

Regional LNs= Plevic (obturator, common/external iliac, lateral sacral, para-aortic) and retroperitoneal LN involvement = T3 and N1

Notes:

Pelvic lymphadenectomy specimen usually contain ≥ 10 LNs

Primary Peritoneal carcinoma staging starts with pT2 (no pT1)

Liver/spleen capsule mets is T3 while liver/spleen parenchymal mets = M1.

Pleural effusion positive cytology = M1.

FIGO staging correspond to TNM

MALE ORGANS

Prostate

T1: Clinically not palpable or visible by imaging

> **T1a:** incidental, ≤5% of tissue resected
> **T1b:** incidental, >5% of tissue resected
> **T1c:** detected by needle bx, after high PSA

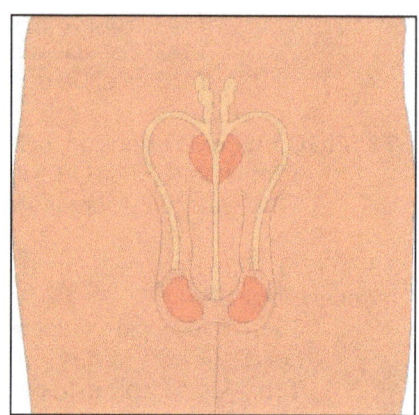

T2: Palpable & Confined within prostate (or apex involvement but intact capsule)

> **T2a:** ≤ ½ of 1 lobe
> **T2b:** > ½ of 1 lobe
> **T2c:** Both lobes

T3: Extra-prostatic extension (<u>**Note**: Invasion into apex or into-but not beyond- prostatic capsule = T2)</u>

> **T3a:** Extracapsular/bladder neck extension (base)
> **T3b:** Seminal vesicle (SV)

T4: Fixed or invades adjacent structures, not SV

N1: Regional LN(s)

Note: Mets ≤ 0.2cm (2mm) = pNmi

M1a: Non-regional LNs

M1b: Bone (s)

M1c: Other site (s)

Note:
- Positive inked (either intra- or extracapsular) margin = R1
- Stage grouping involves PSA level and Gleason score

Clinically important parameters: Gleason 1ry, 2ry and 3ry patterns and No. of positive cores/all cores

Testis

Tis: (Intratubular, germ cell neoplasia in situ = GCNIS)

T1: within testis & epididymis, no LVI

T2: within testis & epididymis **+ LVI** or T. vaginalis invasion (If T. albuginea only= T1)

T3: Spermatic cord ± LVI

T4: Scrotum ± LVI

N1: ≤ 2 cm and or ≤ 5 LNs, none >2cm
N2: >2 -5 cm or >5 LNs, none >5cm or ENE+
N3: > 5 cm
M1a: Non-regional LNs or lung
M1b: Other sites
Serum tumour markers level (S) included in the stage grouping.
Serum Tumour Markers (S)
S0 = normal
S1: LDH < 1.5 X N and hCG : < 5K and AFP : < 1K
S2: LDH 1.5 –10 x N or hCG: 5K–50K or AFP: 1K–10K
S3: LDH > 10 x N or hCG: > 50K or AFP: > 10K

Penis

Ta: Non-invasive verrucous carcinoma
T1a: subepithelial CT (No LVI, not poorly differentiated carcinoma)
T1b: subepithelial CT + LVI OR poorly differentiated carcinoma
T2: corpus spongiosum +/- urethra
T3: corpus cavernosum +/- urethra
T4: adjacent structures.
N1: 1-2 inguinal
N2: >2 inguinal unilat/bilat
N3: pelvic LN (s), unilat/bilat OR ENE of any regional LN
M1: distant mets + LN outside pelvis

Prognostic factors: Grade, HPV Status, p53, HIV, EGFR

URINARY SYSTEM / ADRENAL

Adrenal Cortical Carcinoma

T1: < 5 cm, no extra-adrenal invasion
T2: > 5 cm, no extra-adrenal invasion
T3: Local invasion, but not T4
T4: Adjacent organs (great vessels, kidney, pancreas, liver, spleen, diaphragm)

Kidney

T1: ≤7 cm, within the kidney (**T1a**: ≤4 cm, **T1b** :> 4cm)
T2: >7 cm, within the kidney (**T2a**: >7-10cm, **T2b**: >10cm)
T3: major veins or perinephric/peripelvic fat **(grossly)**
T3a: Renal vein or perinephric/peripelvic fat
T3b: extends to Vena cava < diaphragm
T3c: extends to Vena cava > diaphragm or invades vena cava wall
T4: Beyond Gerota fascia or adrenal (ipsi)
N1: regional LN (s)
Clinically important:
Invasion beyond capsule into fat or peri-sinus tissues, venous involvement, Adrenal Extension, Fuhrman Grade, sarcomatoid features, tumour necrosis

Renal Pelvis, Ureter TCC

Ta: Non-invasive papillary
Tis: In situ
T1: Subepithelial CT
T2: MP
T3: Beyond MP
T4: Adjacent organs/ perinephric fat
N1: Single ≤2 cm
N2: Single >2 - 5 cm or multiple, any <5 cm
N3: Any >5 cm

Urinary bladder TCC

Tis: In situ: "flat T"
Ta: Non-invasive papillary
T1: Subepithelial CT
T2: MP
    T2a: Inner ½,
    T2b: Outer ½
T3: perivesical (beyond muscularis)
    T3a: microscopic
    T3b: macroscopic
T4: Extravesical organs/structures
    T4a: prostatic stroma, SV, uterus, vagina
    T4b: pelvic wall, abdominal wall
N1: 1 LN in true pelvis (obturator, external iliac or pre-sacral LN)
N2: >1 LN in the true pelvis
N3: common iliac LN (s)

M1a Non regional lymph nodes
M1b Other distant metastasis
Prognostic factors:
Superficial TCC (Tis, T1): recurrences, age, smoking, p53, DNA methylation, LVI
Locally advanced TCC (T2-T4): age, margin, histological type and grade, LVI, CIS+, T size, Haemoglobin, response to chemoTx, p53, p63, p21, Rb, Ki67, EGF receptor, HER2 expression, E-cadherin, BRCA1 or MMR mutations. Squamous differentiation is bad.

Urethra and Prostatic Urethra (PU)

Same like bladder for Ta, Tis and T1
T2: Corpus spongiosum, prostate, periurethral muscles
T3: Corpus cavernosum, beyond prostate capsule, anterior vagina (, bladder neck
T4: Other adjacent organs
N1: 1 LN
N2: Multiple LNs

SOFT TISSUE SARCOMA (STS)

Definition: Soft tissue includes all tissue between skin and bone (fat, nerves, muscle, fascia, blood vessels…)

As a part of the staging, histological diagnosis and grading into low/high grade is essential. Some tumours are high grade by definition. Examples include MFH, synovial sarcoma, and soft part alveolar sarcoma

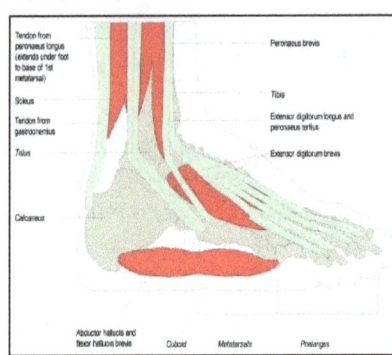

Notes:

- Superficial = all the tumour above superficial facia without invasion to the fascia. Muscle involvement = deep location.
- Stage grouping includes grade.
- STS not included in TNM: Kaposi, angiosarcoma, DFSP (dermatofibrosarcoma protuberans), fibromatosis, GIST and visceral STS (hollow or parenchymatous) or brain

Extremity and Superficial Trunk and retroperitoneum

T1: ≤ 5cm
T2: >5 -10cm
T3: > 10-15cm
T4: >15cm

Head and Neck

T1 ≤ 2cm
T2 >2 -4cm
T3: > 4cm
T4a: orbit, skull base or dura, central compartment viscera, facial skeleton, and or pterygoid muscles
T4b: brain parenchyma, encases the carotid artery, pre-vertebral muscle or CNS by perineural spread

Thoracic and Abdominal Viscera

T1: 1 organ
T2a: serosa or visceral peritoneum invasion
T2b: beyond serosa (microscopic)
T3: another organ OR beyond serosa (macroscopic)
T4a: Multifocal invades ≤ 2 sites in 1 organ
T4b: Multifocal >2-5 sites
T4c: Multifocal > 5 sites

BONE TUMOURS

The staging applies to all primary malignant bone tumours except lymphomas, multiple myeloma, juxtacortical osteosarcoma/ chondrosarcoma.

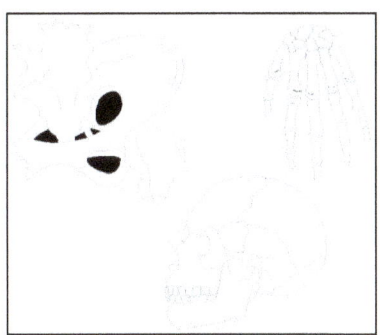

Tumours of limbs, Trunk, Skull and Facial Bones

T1:≤ 8cm,
T2: >8cm,
T3: Discontinuous Ts in primary site
Grade: Low grade, High grade
Stage grouping includes grade (high grade tumours include Ewing's)
Percentage of necrosis following Tx should be included in the report

Tumours of Spine:

A vertebrae have 5 segments:
- Right pedicle
- Right body
- Left body
- Left pedicle
- Posterior element

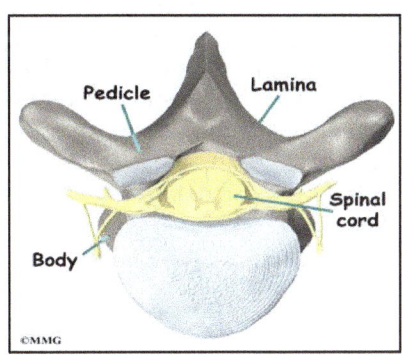

T1: 1-2 adjacent vertebral segment
T2: 3 adjacent vertebral segment
T3: 4 adjacent vertebral segment
T4a: invades spinal canal
T4b: invades adjacent vessels or vascular tumour thrombosis

Tumours of Pelvis

The 4 pelvic segments:
- Sacrum lateral to the sacral foramen
- Iliac wing
- Acetabulum/peri-acetabulum
- Pelvic rami, symphysis and ischium

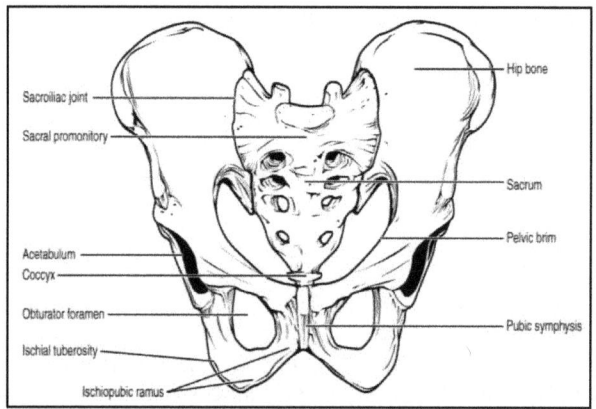

T1a: ≤ 8 cm + 1 segment + no extra-osseus extension (EOE-)
T1b: > 8 cm in size + 1 segment (EOE-)
T2a: ≤ 8 cm + 1 segment (EOE+) OR 2 adjacent segments (EOE-)
T2b: > 8 cm + 1 segment (EOE+) OR 2 adjacent segments (EOE-)
T3a: ≤ 8 cm + 2 segments (EOE+)
T3b: > 8 cm + 2 segments (EOE+)
T4a: 3 adjacent segments or crossing sacroiliac joint to sacral neuro-foramen
T4b: T encasing external iliac vessels OR tumour thrombus in major pelvic vessels

N1: Regional
M1a: Lung, **M1b**: Other sites

Prognostic factors: location, size, extent of disease, tumour response to neoadjuvant chemotherapy, margins, LDH, Alkaline phosphatase

SKIN TUMOURS

Staging applies to:
All sites except Vulva, penis, **eyelid** and head & neck
All tumours except Merkel and melanoma

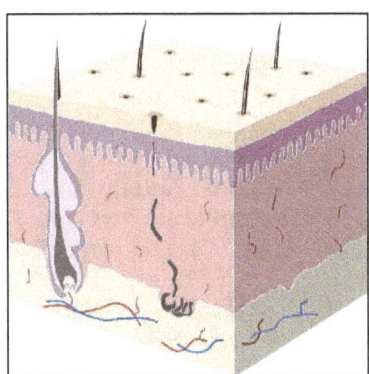

T1: ≤2 cm
T2: > 2 - 4cm
T3: > 4 cm or minor bone erosion or perineural invasion OR deep invasion (SC fat or > 6mm from granular layer of N epid, OR perineural inv clinically)
T4a: gross cortical bone / marrow invasion

T4b: skull base or axial skeleton (including foramina and/or vertebral foramen involvement)
N1: 1 LN ≤ 3 cm
N2: 1 ipsi LN >3 -6 cm, or multiple any ≤6 cm
N3: Any ipsi > 6 cm
If contra LN = M1

Skin Carcinoma of the Head and Neck

T stage is similar to non-Head and neck while nodal stage is same as nodal stage of Oral carcinoma where ENE counts

Merkel cell carcinoma

T1: ≤2 cm,
T2: > 2 -5 cm,
T3: > 5 Cm,
T4: Deep extra-dermal structures (e.g., cartilage, bone, muscle…)
N1a (sn): mets in SLNB
N1a: Mets in LN dissection
N1b: Macroscopic mets (clinically apparent)
N2: In-transit mets (No LN mets)
N3: In-transit mets + LN mets
Note: In-transit mets: discontinuous T away from 1° T , present between 1° T and LN.
M1a: distant Skin, SCT OR non-regional LN
M1b: Lung
M1c: Other site (s)

Melanoma

Tis: in situ, lentigo maligna
pTx includes shave biopsies and regressed melanomas.
T1: ≤1.0 mm in thickness
    T1a: ≤ 0.8mm, no ulcer
    T1b: ≤ 0.8mm + ulcer or > 0.8-1mm +/- ulcer
T2: > 1-2mm (T2a: no ulcer, **T2b:** + ulcer)
T3: >2-4mm (T3a: no ulcer, **T3b:** + ulcer)
T4: >4mm (T4a: no ulcer, **T4b:** + ulcer)

N1: 1LN (**N1a:** micro, **N1b:** macro)
N2: 2-3 LNs (**N2a:** micro, **N2b:** macro, **N2c:** satellite/in-transit + no LN mets)
N3: ≥4LN or matted or satellite/in-transit + LN mets
Note: Satellites are T nodules (macro or micro) within 2 cm of 1° T. In-transit mets involves skin or SCT (subcutaneous tissue)> 2 cm from 1° T but not beyond the regional LNs.
M1a: distant skin/SCT, or distant LNs
M1b: lung
M1c: any site (not CNS)
M1d: CNS
Prognostic factors for melanoma: T stage, mitotic rate, metastatic disease, tumour infiltrating lymphocytes (TIL), regression, immunosuppressive use, LVI, perineural invasion, site, Family Hx, female-better, younger-better

CLARKE'S STAGING: Tumour Growth-Phase
Stage I: Melanoma in situ, limited to epidermis.
Stage II: Radial-Growth-Phase. T invaded papillary dermis.
Stage III: Vertical-Growth-Phase. T invaded reticular dermis.
Stage IV: Vertical-Growth-Phase. T invaded beyond reticular dermis.
Stage V: Subcutaneous invasion, metastases.

Primary cutaneous lymphoma

T1: patches/ plaques, <10% of skin (**T1a**: patch, **T1b**: plaque).
T2: patches /plaques, > 10% of skin (**T2a**: patch, **T2b**: plaque).
T3: ≥ 1 tumour (s) (≥1cm)
T4: confluent erythema ≥80% skin surface

N1: Clinically abn. LNs, Dutch grade 1 (clone -/+). (T-cell clonality is determined by PCR or Southern blot analysis of receptor gene)
N2: Clinically abn LNs Dutch grade 2 (clone -/+)
N3: Clinically abn LNs, Dutch grades 3-4 (clone -/+)
M1: visceral involvement histologically

Peripheral blood involvement (B): included in stage grouping
B0: Not significant: ≤ 5% Sézary cells (clone -/+)
B1: Low blood tumour burden: > 5% Sézary cells but not B2 (clone -/+)
B2: High blood tumour burden: ≥1000/µL Sézary cells with clone+

EYE- OPHTHALMIC TUMOURS

Carcinoma of Skin of the Eyelid

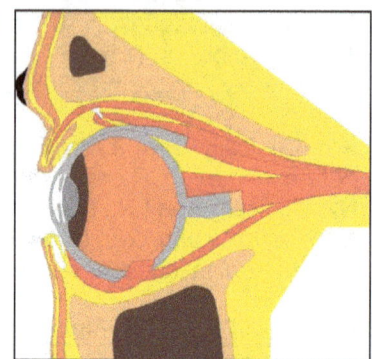

T1: ≤ 10mm
>**T1a**: not tarsal plate or lid margin
>**T1b**: not tarsal plate or lid margin
>**T1c**: full thickness of eyelid

T2: >10-20mm
>**T1a**: not tarsal plate or lid margin
>**T1b**: not tarsal plate or lid margin
>**T1c**: full thickness of eyelid

T3: Tumour > 20 mm
>**T1a**: not tarsal plate or lid margin
>**T1b**: not tarsal plate or lid margin
>**T1c**: full thickness of eyelid

T4: adjacent ocular, or orbital, or facial structures
>**T4a**: ocular or intraorbital structures
>**T4b**: bony walls of orbit or paranasal sinuses or lacrimal sac/nasolacrimal duct or brain

N1: 1 LN, ipsi, ≤3 cm
N2: 1 LN, ipsi, >3 cm, or bilat or contra LNs

Conjunctival carcinoma

T1: ≤5 mm, invades BM
T2: > 5 mm, invades BM
T3: adjacent structures (Not orbit)
T4: orbit +/- further extension
>**T4a**: orbit soft tissue
>**T4b**: orbit bone
>**T4c**: paranasal sinuses
>**T4d**: brain

Conjunctival Melanoma

Tis: in situ
T1: bulbar conj
>**T1a:** ≤2mm T thickness + inv. of subst propria
>**T1b:** >2mm + inv. of subst propria

T2: non bulbar conj (forniceal, palpebral or tarsal) + inv of Caruncle
>**T2a:** ≤2mm T thickness + inv of subst propria
>**T2b:** >2mm + inv. of subst propria

T3: any size + local invasion
      T3a: eye, **T3b:** eyelid, **T3c:** orbit, **T3d:** sinus
T4: **any size + CNS invasion**

UVEAL Melanoma

Iris
T1: within iris
T1a: ≤ 3 o'clock, **T1b:** > 3 o'clock, **T1c:** + glaucoma
T2: ciliary body/choroid:
      T2a: ciliary body, no glaucoma
      T2b: choroid, no glaucoma
      T2c: ciliary or choroid + glaucoma
T3: sclera
T4: extra-ocular (extra scleral)
T4a: ≤5mm, **T4b:** >5mm

Ciliary body/choroid

There are 4 tumour size categories based on tumour thickness and tumour diameter (complex issue, clinical). Examples:
Size category 1: tumour thickness 3mm and diameter 3mm
Size category 2: tumour thickness 6mm and diameter 6mm
Size category 3: tumour thickness 9mm and diameter 12mm
Size category 4: tumour thickness > 15mm and diameter >18mm
T1: category 1
T1a: No ciliary or extra-ocular, **T1b:** ciliary only **T1c:** extra-ocular ≤5mm, **T1d**: ciliary +extra-ocular ≤5mm
T2: category 2
T2a: No ciliary or extra-ocular, **T2b:** ciliary only **T2c:** extra-ocular ≤5mm, **T2d**: ciliary +extra-ocular ≤5mm
T3: category3
T3a: No ciliary or extra-ocular, **T3b:** ciliary only **T3c:** extra-ocular ≤5mm, **T3d**: ciliary +extra-ocular ≤5mm
T4: category4
T4a: No ciliary or extra-ocular, **T4b:** ciliary only **T4c:** extra-ocular ≤5mm, **T4d**: ciliary +extra-ocular ≤5mm, **T4e**: Any tumour size category + extraocular extension > 5 mm in

Retinoblastoma

There are pTNM and cTNM. Only pTNM discussed
T1: confined to eye, no optic n or choroidal inv

T2: intra-ocular inv.

T2a: Focal choroidal inv + pre or intralaminar inv of the optic n
T2b: stroma of iris and/or trabecular meshwork and/or Schlemm's canal

T3: significant optic n/choroidal invasion

T3a: choroidal inv > 3mm or multiple inv totalling >3mm or full thickness inv
T3b: Retrolaminar inv of optic n without inv of transected end of optic n
T3c: Partial thickness inv. of sclera within inner 2/3
T3d: Full thickness inv. into outer 1/3 of sclera and/or inv into or around emissary channels

T4: extra-ocular : inv. optic n at transected end, in meningeal space around the optic n, full thickness invasion of the sclera + inv of episclera, adipose tissue, extra-ocular muscle, bone, conjunctiva, or eyelid.

M1a Single or multiple mets to sites other than CNS
M1b Mets to CNS parenchyma or CSF fluid

Lacrimal gland carcinoma-Meibomian carcinoma

T1: ≤2 cm, +/- extra-gland extension to orbital soft tissue
    T1a: no periosteal or bone inv
    T1b: periosteal, no bone inv
    T1c: bone inv
T2: > 2 - 4 cm, limited to lacrimal gland
    T2a: no periosteal or bone inv
    T2b: periosteal, no bone inv
    T2c: bone inv
T3: > 4 cm + extraglandular extension to orbital soft tissue
    T3a: no periosteal or bone inv
    T3b: periosteal, no bone inv
    T3c: bone inv
T4: adjacent structures (sinuses, temporal fossa, pterygoid fossa, sup orbital fissure, cavernous sinus, and/or brain):
    T4a: ≤ 2cm
    T4b: >2-4cm
    T4c: > 4 cm

Orbital sarcoma

T1: ≤20 mm
T2: >20 mm, not T3 or T4

T3: orbital tissues and/or bony walls
T4: globe or periorbital tissue (eyelids, temporal fossa, nose, sinuses, or CNS)

Ocular adnexal lymphoma

T1: within conjunctiva. No orbital involvement
    T1a: bulbar conj
    T1b: palpebral conj
    T1c: extensive conj involvement
T2: orbit
    T2a: anterior orbit
    T2b: anterior orbit + lacrimal
    T2c: posterior orbit
    T2d: naso-lacrimal drainage system
T3: pre-septal eyelid
T4: beyond orbit to adjacent structures
    T4a: nasopharynx
    T4b: bone (including periosteum)
    T4c: sinuses (maxillofacial, ethmoidal or frontal)
    T4d: Intracranial

HODGKIN'S AND NON- HODGKIN'S LYMPHOMA

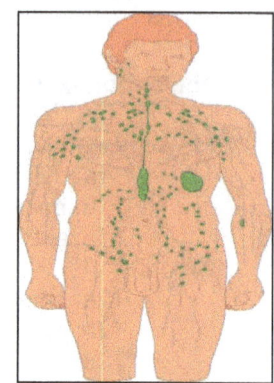

(Lugano modification of ANN ARBOR classification), clinical staging

Lymphatic and Extra-lymphatic Disease
The lymphatic organs are: LNs, Waldeyer ring (oral), Spleen, Appendix, Thymus, Peyer patches

Clinical Stages (CS)

Limited Stage

Stage I
1 LN region (I)
Localized 1 extra-lymphatic organ (I_E)

Stage II
≥2 LN regions, same side of diaphragm (II)
Localized 1 extra-lymphatic organ + its regional LN, ± other LN regions same side of diaphragm (II_E)

Bulky Stage II
Stage II +1LN > 10 cm OR > 1/3 of thoracic diameter on CT.

Advanced Stage

Stage III
LN regions both sides of diaphragm (III) ± Spleen (III_S)

Stage IV
Disseminated (non-localised involvement) ≥1 extra-lymphatic organ(s) ± it's associated LN (s) OR 1 extra-lymphatic + separate LNs, same or both sides of diaphragm. (Liver involvement is usually IV)

All stages divided into:
A. No weight loss/fever/sweats
B. Weight loss>10%/fever >38°C/night sweats
Bulky stage II >6 cm in follicular lymphoma, >10 cm in diffuse large cell lymphoma.

PAEDIATRIC TUMOURS

Hepatoblastoma, Osteosarcoma, Ewing Sarcoma

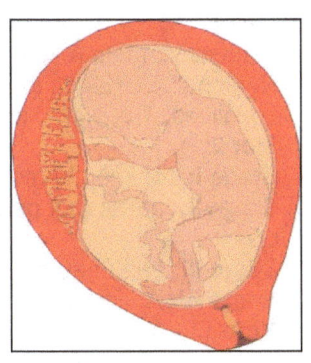

Tier 1 & 2
Metastatic: metastases present
Localized: 1ry Tumour +/- regional LNs

Rhabdomyosarcoma
Tier 1
Like tier 1 & 2 for hepatoblastoma
Tier 2
Favourable or Unfavourable anatomic site determine prognosis. See below
T1: 1 anatomic site
       T1a: ≤ 5 cm
       T1b: >5 cm
T2: beyond anatomic site
       T2a: ≤ 5 cm
       T2b: >5 cm
Favourable: H&N (except para-meningeal) and genitourinary (except bladder & prostate)
Unfavourable: Any other sites

Soft Tissue Sarcoma (Not Rhabdomyosarcoma)

Tier 1
Like tier 1 & 2 for hepatoblastoma
Tier 2
TNM of adults

Ovary

Tier 1
Metastatic: mets (except peritoneal)
Regional: T extends to pelvis, peritoneum, or retroperitoneal LNs
Localised: T confined to ovaries (1 or both)
Tier 2
Stage I: confined to ovaries (1 or both)
Stage II: pelvis (not peritoneum outside the pelvis) nor to retroperitoneal LNs
Stage III: peritoneum outside the pelvis and/or retroperitoneal LNs
Stage IV: Any mets (except peritoneal)
Note
TNM = FIGO stage.

Testes

Tier 1
Like tier 1 & 2 for hepatoblastoma
Tier 2
 Like TNM of adults

Wilms Tumour- Nephroblastoma

Tier 1
Like tier 1 & 2 for hepatoblastoma
Tier 2
2 staging classifications based on ChemoTx
- **No prior Chemo:** National Wilms Tumour Study Group (NWTSG) classification
- **Prior Chemo:** International Society of Paediatric Oncology (SIOP) classification

SIOP Classification of Childhood Renal Tumours:
>**I – Low Risk:**
>>Mesoblastic nephroma (5% of tumours)
>>Nephroblastoma- cystic/ necrotic
>
>**II - Intermediate Risk:**
>>Nephroblastoma subtypes: epithelial/ stromal/ mixed/ regressive/ focally anaplastic
>
>**III – High Risk:**
>>Nephroblastoma- blastema/ diffusely anaplastic
>>Clear cell sarcoma (4%), Rhabdoid tumour (2%)

Notes:
- Renal Ts in children are removed after neoadjuvant ChemoTx so tumour necrosis is due to effect of ChemoTx. % of viable vs. non-viable tumour cells reflects tumour response.
- Renal sinus known microscopically by absence of renal capsule, and presence of vessels and nerves + fat.
- % of anaplastic component in the nephroblastoma should be calculated.

Staging (Abdominal staging) of Nephroblastoma (Wilms):

I: limited to kidney (and renal capsule)
II: beyond kidney but clear resection margin
III: At resection margin, capsule ruptured, abdominal LN mets, peritoneum involved or previous wedge bx
IV: mets, or to non-abdominal LNs
V: bilateral tumours

Retinoblastoma

Tier1
Like tier 1 & 2 for hepatoblastoma
Localized Intraocular
Tier2
Only after enucleation (pathological classification).
Prognostic factors
Stage 0: confined to the globe. No enucleation
pStage I Enucleation + negative margins (R0)
pStage II Enucleation + microscopic residual disease (R1)
pStage III Involvement of the orbit and/or metastases to regional LNs
cStage IV Metastatic disease

Hodgkin & Non- Hodgkin's Lymphoma

Tier 1
Advanced: Involvement of bone marrow and/or CNS
Limited: No involvement of bone marrow or CNS
Tier 2
Stage I
1 tumour mass or nodal area, (except mediastinum & abdomen)
Stage II
1tumour mass + regional LN (s) or ≥ 2 tumours and/or nodal regions on same side of the diaphragm, OR resected 1° GIT tumour +/- regional LN (s)

Stage III
Tumours and /or LNs on opposite sides of diaphragm OR
1° intrathoracic OR extensive 1° intra-abdominal OR para-spinal OR
epidural
Stage IV
Bone marrow and/or CNS

Medulloblastoma and Ependymoma

Tier 1
Metastatic: Disease beyond local site
Localized: Localized disease
Tier 2
Based on the extent of metastatic disease

NEUROBLASTOMA

Tier 1
Localized: confined to 1o site (no vital organs invasion).
Loco-regional: More extensive without metastatic disease
MS: Metastatic confined to skin, liver and/or bone marrow in a patient
< 18 months of age
Metastatic: mets in sites not mentioned in MS
Tier 2
International Neuroblastoma Risk Group Staging System (INRGSS)

OTHER ORGANS/TUMOURS STAGING NOT INCLUDED IN TNM8

Adult Brain tumours

No staging of brain tumours in TNM8, because of inherent inability of brain tumours to mets and lack of lymphatics in the brain. Previously published TNM:

Supratentorial
T1:<5 cm unilat, **T2:** >5 cm, unilat
Infratentorial
T1: <3 cm unilat, **T2:** >3 cm, unilat
For both
T3: Invades ventricular system
T4: crosses midline or invades infra- (or supra-) tentorially
Grading involved in stage grouping. Grading parameters: necrosis, mitosis and cellularity

Phyllodes tumour of the breast

Phyllodes tumour of the breast is divided into benign, borderline or malignant based on the stromal overgrowth (>40x without epithelium), mitosis (>10/10hpf), stromal atypia or heterologous elements. Metastasis reported in regional lymph nodes in 5% of cases and hematogenous spread occurs mainly to the lung. No TNM staging for malignant or borderline tumours.

Haggitt levels for invasion in a pedunculated polyp:

- **Level 1**: inv. within head of the polyp
- **Level 2**: inv. into junction of head and stalk
- **Level 3**: inv. into stalk
- **Level 4**: inv. in SM below stalk

Kikuchi levels for submucosal (sm) invasion in sessile polyp:

- **Sm1**: minor SM invasion from MM to depth of 300 μm
- **Sm2**: intermediate invasion.
- **Sm3**: invasion near inner surface of MP

IB. NON-CANCER STAGING

PRIMARY BILIARY CIRRHOSIS-PBC

I.   Florid duct lesions or portal hepatitis
II. Ductular reaction or periportal hepatitis
III. Bridging/septal fibrosis or bridging necrosis
IV. Cirrhosis

PRIMARY SCLEROSING CHOLANGITIS-PSC

I.   Cholangitis / portal hepatitis
II. Periportal fibrosis or periportal hepatitis
III. Bridging fibrosis or necrosis
IV. Cirrhosis

LIVER FIBROSIS STAGE

Stage 0, none
Stage 1, perivenular (zone 3) fibrosis
Stage 2, perivenular + portal fibrosis
Stage 3, bridging fibrosis
Stage 4, cirrhosis

II.PATHOLOGICAL GRADING

IIA. CANCER GRADING

IIB.BCANCER RESPONSE GRADING

IIC.NON-CANCER GRADING

IIA. CANCER GRADING

Grading of a tumour is done based on tumour differentiation (differentiation = resemblance of the tumour to tissue of origin)

Grading includes assessment of both the architectural and cytologic features of the tumour.
- Combined architecture and cytology: most of tumours
- Pure architecture grading: Gleason's in prostate
- Nuclear grading: RCC, DCIS

Grading is included in tumour staging in brain tumours
High-grade tumours require wider excision, has high rate of recurrence and poor prognosis
Low grade = well differentiated= grade 1
High grade = poorly differentiated= grade 3

TUMOURS OF MULTIPLE ORGANS

ADENOCARCINOMA

Grade 1, Well differentiated, low grade: >95% of T composed of glands
Grade 2, Moderately differentiated: 50%- 95% of T composed of glands
Grade 3: Poorly differentiated, high grade: 5% to 49% of T composed of glands
Grade 4, anaplastic: <5% of T composed of glands

SQUAMOUS CELL CARCINOMA

Sites: oral, skin, oesophagus, lung, cervix, vulva, vagina, penis, UB

- **G1, Well differentiated, low grade**: nests of squamous + prominent cell borders+ keratin pearl formation (in keratinizing type)
- **G2, Moderately differentiated, intermediate grade**: small nests of squamous cells + moderate pleomorphism
- **G3, Poorly differentiated, high grade**: sheets of anaplastic cells + severe pleomorphism + ill-defined cell borders.

Variants of Squamous Cell Carcinoma

High-grade variants
    Spindle /sarcomatoid
    Basaloid
    Small cell
    Lymphoepithelioma-like
Low-grade variants
    Verrucous
    Papillary
    Adenoid

NEUROENDOCRINE TUMOURS

Neuroendocrine markers used to define neuroendocrine tumours (Synaptophysin, Chromogranin and CD56), however Ki67 proliferation index is required for grading (in addition to morphology) for pancreatic and GI neuroendocrine tumours (NETs)

G1: (well differentiated, low grade, carcinoid): Ki-67 index <3%
G2: (intermediate grade, atypical carcinoid): Ki-67 index 3- 20%
G3: (poorly differentiated, high grade, NE carcinoma): Ki-67 index >20%

HEAD AND NECK TUMOURS

ADENOID CYSTIC CARCINOMA-Salivary gland

Low grade. Tubular pattern
Intermediate grade. Cribriform pattern
High grade. Solid pattern

MUCOEPIDERMOID CARCINOMA-MEC-

MEC is characterised by cords or sheets of different proportions of mucous, squamous, intermediate and clear cells

TWO GRADES:
- **Low grade**: mucinous and intermediate cells with bland nuclei form glandular spaces

- **High grade**: solid and infiltrative growth pattern of atypical epidermoid and intermediate cells with cytoplasmic clearing and small number of mucinous cells; < 20% intracystic component

AFIP point system:

- 2 points if < 20% intracystic component
- 2 points if neural invasion
- 3 points if necrosis
- 3 points if 4+ mitotic figures/10 HPF
- 4 points if anaplasia

Low grade if total score is 0 - 4 points, intermediate grade if 5 - 6 points, high grade if 7+ points

GENITAL (MALE/FEMALE) TUMOURS

PROSTATE ADENOCARCINOMA

GLEASON GRADING AND GLEASON SCORE

Gleason score is between 2 -10 and it is the sum of primary (most prevalent grade) and secondary pattern (worst grade)

GLEASON PATTERNS (GRADES)

Gleason grade 1: well circumscribed nodules of single, separate glands. Not diagnosed in needle biopsies
Gleason grade 2: as grade 1 but some variabilities in gland size. Not diagnosed in needle biopsies
Gleason grade 3: Single, separate, variable glands, irregularly separated, ragged, poorly defined edge.
Gleason grade 4: fused/cribriform glands. Ductal carcinoma is grade 4
Gleason grade 5: either single cells with no glands or comedo pattern

DIFFERENTIATION GRADES:
- Gleason ≤ 6 Well differentiated, G1
- Gleason 7 Moderately differentiated, G2
- Gleason 8-10 Poorly differentiated/undifferentiated, G3

WHO GRADE GROUPS BASED ON GLEASON SCORE:
Group 1: 3+3
Group 2: 3+4
Group 3: 4+3
Group 4: 4+4
Group 5: 4+5, 5+4 or 5+5

PENILE / VULVAL INTRAEPITHELIAL NEOPLASIA (PEIN, VIN)

PEIN1/ VIN 1, mild squamous dysplasia, lower 1/3
PEIN2/VIN 2, moderate squamous dysplasia, lower 2/3
PEIN/3/VIN 3, severe squamous dysplasia/carcinoma in situ, full thickness

3 markers need to be emplpyed p16, p53, Ki67

CERVICAL INTRAEPITHELIAL NEOPLSIA (CIN)

CIN 1, mild squamous dysplasia, +/-HPV related changes (koilocytic changes, raisinoid nuclei)
CIN 2, moderate squamous dysplasia, lower 2/3
CIN 3, severe squamous dysplasia, full thickness, +/- squamous metaplastic crypts (glands).

ENDOMETRIOID ADENOCARCINOMA:

Based on % of non-squamous or non-morular -NS/NM- solid glandular growth pattern:
G1= ≤5%
G2= 6-50%
G3= > 50%
Marked nuclear atypia increases the grade by 1.
Serous, clear cell, and mixed mesodermal tumours = Grade 3.

SERTOLI –LEYDIG CELL TUMOUR (SLCT)

Differentiation between Sertoli and Leydig cells in SLCT can be done in well differentiated but difficult in poorly differentiated.
Sertoli cells: columnar + oval grooved nuclei arranged in tubules
Leydig cells: round nuclei + abundant eosinophilic cytoplasm + Reinke crystals + lipofuscin pigment arranged in groups

- ○ **Well differentiated**: Sertoli cell tubules + intervening Leydig cells. No atypia or mitosis
- ○ **Moderately differentiated**: Sertoli cells: tubules or sheets + mixed with Leydig cells. Mild-moderate atypia & mitosis 5 /10hpf.
- ○ **Poorly differentiated**: sarcomatoid sheets of Sertoli cells. Few or no Leydig cells. Moderate – severe atypia. Mitosis 20 /10hpf

LEYDIG CELL TUMOUR

Benign, unless there are features of malignancy, including: atypical mitosis, mitoses > 3/10hpf, Infiltrating tumour edge, Invasion of rete testis, necrosis or tumour vascular emboli

IMMATURE /MALIGNANT TERATOMA

Immature neuroepithelium is the only tissue used in grading. Immature neuroepithelium (spindled or rosettes), formed of cells with little cytoplasm, hyperchromatic nuclei and excess mitoses
Old grading (3 tier)
- Grade 1: < 1 low power field (40x) in any slide
- Grade 2 (high grade): ≥ 1 but < 3 low power fields in any slide
- Grade 3 (high grade): ≥ 3 low power fields in any slide
New grading: (2 tier)
- Low grade: < 1 low power field (40x) in any slide
- High grade: ≥ 1 low power field in any slide

If teratoma has <3mm admixed foci of YS or embryonal ca, no change in grading or prognosis

BREAST TUMOURS

BREAST DUCTAL CARCINOMA IN SITU

This is a nuclear grading system

Grade 1. The nuclei are small, round, and uniform, less than 1.5 times the size of an RBC.

Grade 2. Larger nuclei, 1.5- 2 times the size of an RBC, few mitoses

Grade 3. Large nuclei > 2.5 times the size of an RBC, prominent nucleoli, and frequent mitoses

BREAST CARCINOMA GRADING

Elston / Nottingham modification of Bloom-Richardson system. The system assess three parameters:

Tumour tubule formation:
1 point: > 75% of tumour
2 points: 10 - 75% of tumour
3 points: < 10% of tumour

Mitotic count/10hpf

1 point:: 0 - 9

2 points: 10 - 19

3 points: 20+

Nuclear pleomorphism:
1 point: mild
2 points: moderate
3 points: severe

Final Scoring
3 - 5 points: Grade 1
6 - 7 points; Grade 2
8 - 9 points: Grade 3

SUBTYPING OF BREAST CARCINOMA

A. *In situ* carcinoma

- Ductal: cribriform, solid, comedo…etc
- Lobular

B. Invasive carcinoma
- Classic ductal, not otherwise specified (NOS). Most common
- Lobular: classic, pleomorphic, solid, alveolar
- Metaplastic
- Invasive cribriform
- Colloid/mucinous
- Lymphoepithelioma-like
- Medullary
- Tubular
- Neuroendocrine
- Inflammatory
- Papillary
- Micropapillary
- Myoepithelial
- Apocrine
- Oncocytic
- Others : Cystic hypersecretory, Adenosquamous, Glycogen rich, Lipid rich, Secretory, Small cell, Squamous cell, Adenoid cystic, Basal cell, Mucinous cystadenocarcinoma, Mucoepidermoid, Central necrotizing, Tubulolobular, Mixed

RENAL CELL CARCINOMA

Fuhrman grading system is a nuclear grading system uses the low magnification power to grade the nuclei in the worst area of the tumour

Fuhrman's grading system is used for **clear cell and papillary** renal cell carcinomas

Fuhrman Nuclear Grade:
Grade 1: Nuclei: round, uniform. No nucleoli
Grade 2: Nuclei: slightly irregular. Nucleoli: visible at high-power x400
Grade 3: Nuclei: very irregular outlines. Nucleoli: visible at x 100
Grade 4: Nuclei: Bizarre and multilobed, spindle. Nucleoli: Prominent. Cells may be sarcomatoid or rhabdoid

Leibovich (Mayo) score: (low/ intermediate/ high risk group)

•Pathological T stage 0-4
•Nodal status: 0-2
•Tumour size:
>   <10cm = 0
>   >10cm = 1
•Nuclear Grade: 0-3
•Histological tumour necrosis: 0-1

Total Scores range from 0 –11
  - Low=0-2
  - Intermediate =3-5
  - High= 6 or more

HEPATOCELLULAR CARCINOMA

Classic HCC graded as

- Well-differentiated HCC. Minimal cytologic atypia, trabecular or pseudoglandular.
- Moderately differentiated HCC. Moderate atypia, psudoglandular + well-defined nucleoli.
- Poorly differentiated HCC. Pleomorphic tumour cells +/- giant cells, solid nests.

FOLLICULAR LYMPHOMA

According to WHO classification, follicular lymphoma is graded according to number of centroblasts in 10 neoplastic follicles, per hpf. Centroblasts are large non-cleaved cells with 1-3 nucleoli attached to the inner nuclear membrane
Grade 1. 0–5 centroblasts/hpf.
Grade 2. 6–15 centroblasts/hpf.
Grade 3. >15 centroblasts/hpf.

THYMUS TUMOURS

Thymic tumours are classified into

- **Well-Differentiated** (Thymoma): Like normal thymus + No significant cytological atypia in the tumour cells.
- **Moderately Differentiated** Thymic Epithelial Neoplasm (Atypical Thymoma): Partial loss of normal thymus appearance, + moderate cytologic atypia.
- **Poorly Differentiated** Thymic Epithelial Neoplasm (Thymic Carcinoma): Prominent cytologic atypia present

BRAIN AND NEURAL TUMOURS

GLIOMAS/ASTROCYTIC TUMOURS

WHO grading system
Grade1, fibrillary astrocytoma, pilocytic astrocytoma and subependymal giant cell astrocytoma: mild cellularity, no necrosis, no vascular proliferation, no mitoses.
Grade 2, well-differentiated/diffuse astrocytoma: moderate cellularity mild to moderate atypia, rare mitoses, no vascular proliferation or necrosis.
Grade 3, anaplastic/malignant astrocytoma, moderate to high cellularity severe atypia, frequent mitoses. e.g., gemistocytic astrocytoma.
Grade 4: Glioblastoma Multiforme: Necrosis and vascular proliferation + frequent mitoses and severe pleomorphism.

OLFACTORY NEUROBLASTOMA

Hyams grading system:
Grade1: Prominent lobulation, prominent neurofibrillary background, high number of rosettes, mild pleomorphism, few mitosis, no necrosis, calcification

Grade4: no lobulation, no neurofibrillary background, no rosettes, severe pleomorphism, excess mitoses, excess necrosis, no rosettes, no calcification

Grade 2&3 intermediate between 1&4

SOFT TISSUE TUMOURS

French Federation of Cancer Centres **Sarcoma** Group **{FNCLCC}** **grading system for soft tissue sarcoma (STS):**

Tumour differentiation:
1= STS resembling adult mesenchyme, e.g., liposarcoma
2= STS where histologic type is certain, e.g., myxoid liposarcoma
3= embryonal/undifferentiated/uncertain origin, e.g., osteosacroma, Ewing's sarcoma, synovial, PNET

Mitotic count:
1= 0-9/10hpf
2= 10-19/10hpf
3= ≥20/10hpf

Tumour necrosis:
1=No necrosis
2=<50%
3= ≥50%

Final Score:
Grade 1= 2 or 3
Grade 2= 4 or 5
Grade3= 6, 7 or 8

IIB. CANCER RESPONSE GRADING

COLORECTAL (POST-NEOADJUVANT THERAPY):

Tumour regression grading (TRG) evaluates the response of a malignant tumour to preoperative chemo/radiotherapy in colorectal cancer

TRG4: total regression of the tumour, no viable tumour cells (tumour ablation). The tumour mass becomes totally necrotic or fibrosed.

TRG3: fibrosis/necrosis occupies most of the residual tumour mass (>50% tumour regression)

TRG2: dominant tumour with fibrosis/necrosis in 25-50% of the tumour mass

TRG1: minor regression, fibrosis/necrosis in <25% of the tumour mass

TRG0: no regression (chemo/radio-resistant tumour)

BREAST RESIDUAL CANCER BURDEN:

Residual Cancer Burden (RCB) measures residual disease after neoadjuvant chemotherapy (NAC).

RCB-0: Pathological complete response   (pCR)

RCB-1: Partial response (minimal residual disease, <10% tumour remains in tumour bed)

RCB-2: Partial response (significant tumour remaining, >10% tumour remains in tumour bed)

RCB-3: No evidence of response

Residual Cancer Burden (RCB) involved assessment of two parameters (cellularity of residual tumour cells in tumour bed and number + size of LN mets):

A. Tumour response
Complete response: either
    (i) No residual tumour
    (ii) No residual invasive tumour but DCIS present.
Partial response: either
    (i) <10% of residual tumour
    (ii) 10–50% of residual tumour
    (iii) >50% of residual tumour
No response.

B. Nodal response
-No nodal mets
-No mets, but fibrosis present (evidence of response)
-Mets + fibrosis
-Mets + No fibrosis.

Alternative way of response assessment is the Miller-Payne system for grading response after neoadjuvant chemotherapy treated breast cancers:

Grade 1: No change
Grade 2: <30% loss of tumour cells
Grade 3: 30% - 90% loss of tumour cells
Grade 4: > 90% loss of tumuor cells
Grade 5: No malignant cells, however, DCIS may be present

The Miller-Payne system does not include lymph nodes response.

IIC. NON CANCER GRADING

GRADING OF NON ALCOHOLIC STEATOHEPATITIS (NASH)-NON ALCOHOLIC FATTY LIVER DISEASE (NAFLD)

Valuation of macrovesicular steatosis using low magnification (4x or lower) Disease severity is assessed separately by grade of activity and stage of fibrosis

ACTIVITY GRADE = non-alcoholic fatty liver disease activity score (NAS) using the sum of 3 components (total 0 - 8 points)

I.   Steatosis
0: < 5%
1: 5 - 33%
2: 34 - 66%
3: > 66%)

II.   Lobular inflammation
0: none
1: < 2 foci/20x field;
2: 2 - 4 foci/20x field
3: > 4 foci/20x field

III.   Ballooning degeneration
0: none
1: few
2: many

Final score:
Total: < 4, non-diagnostic of NAFLD
Total: 5 or more diagnostic of NAFLD

FIBROSIS STAGE
Stage 0, none
Stage 1, perivenular (zone 3) fibrosis
Stage 2, perivenular + portal fibrosis
Stage 3, bridging fibrosis
Stage 4, cirrhosis

METHOTREXATE INDUCED LIVER DISEASE

Grade 1: mild fatty change + mild portal inflammation
Grade 2: G1 + focal necrosis
Grade 3a: G2 + Mild portal fibrosis
Grade 3b: interface hepatitis or bridging fibrosis
Grade 4: cirrhosis

GRADING OF LIVER IRON OVERLOAD IN HAEMOCHROMATOSIS/SIDEROSIS

HISTOLOGIC GRADING OF IRON ACCUMULATION				
0	1+	2+	3+	4+
No stainable iron	Iron in acinar zone 1	Iron in acinar zones 1 & 2	Iron in acinar zones 1, 2, & 3	Iron in all acinar zones & in biliary epithelium

BANFF SCORES FOR ACUTE HEPATIC CELLULAR REJECTION:

Portal inflammation:
Score 1: lymphocytes in some portal tracts
Score 2: lymphocytes+ neutrophils + eosinophils in most portal tracts
Score 3: Score 2 + spill over into peri-portal hepatocytes
Bile duct:
Score1: few bile ducts infiltrated by inflammatory cells
Score 2: all bile ducts infiltrated by inflammatory cells +   cellular atypia in some bile ducts
Score 3: cellular atypia in all bile ducts

Endothelial inflammation:
Score 1: sub-endothelial lymphocytic infiltrate in venules in some portal tracts
Score 2: score 1 but in most portal tracts
Score 3: as score 2 + perivascular inflammation and necrosis

Final score
<3 not diagnostic of rejection
4-5   mild
6-7   moderate
8-9   severe

GRADING OF REJECTION IN HEART TRANSPLANT

Myocardial biopsy most sensitive indicator of rejection Need at least 4 pieces of tissue with myocardium

0: No rejection
I: Mild rejection

> IA: Patchy, perivascular inflammation
> IB: Diffuse, sparse interstitial infiltrate

II: Moderate rejection: Single focus of aggressive infiltrate, and/or isolated myocyte dropout
III: Moderate rejection
> IIIA: Multifocal aggressive interstitial infiltrates
> IIIB: Diffuse inflammation with necrosis

IV: Severe rejection: abundant myocyte death with vasculitis, hemorrhage, neutrophils, necrosis; usually not reversible

GRADING OF PULMONARY HYPERTENSION

> Grades I-III --- reversible
> Grades IV-VI ---- irreversible

- Grade I: Media hypertrophy of small arteries (media thickness > 7% of external diameter of artery
- Grade II: Media hypertrophy + intimal proliferation in small arteries
- Grade III: Concentric intimal fibrosis of small arteries + reduplicated internal elastic lamina +Larger elastic arteries atherosclerosis
- Grade IV: Widespread dilatation of the small arteries and arterioles (+Plexiform lesions)
- Grade V: Above changes + vein-like branches of hypertrophied muscular arteries with minimal media
- Grade VI: Angiomatoid lesions

LUPUS NEPHRITIS GRADING/STAGING/CLASSIFICATION

Renal Pathology Society (RPS) classification of Lupus Nephritis LN (2004)

The below classification determines the prognosis of Lupus disease. Also renal bx in patient with LE is one of the priority biopsies in Pathology Lab.
Classes

I: Minimal Mesangial Lupus Nephritis:
II: Mesangial Proliferative Lupus Nephritis:
III: Focal Lupus Nephritis
IV: Diffuse Lupus Nephritis
V: Membranous Lupus Nephritis
VI: Advanced Sclerosing Lupus Nephritis

Activity index: (max 24 points)

The following are scored based on severity from 0-3

- Glomerular endocapillary proliferation
- Glomerular neutrophilic infiltration
- Wire-loop deposits and hyaline thrombi
- Glomerular fibrinoid necrosis and karyorrhexis
- Cellular crescents
- Interstitial inflammation

Chronicity index: (max 12 points)

The following are scored based on severity from 0-3

- Glomerular sclerosis
- Fibrous crescents
- Tubular atrophy
- Interstitial fibrosis

MISCELLANEOUS SUBJECTS

TUMOUR PROGNOSIS AND PATIENT'S SURVIVAL ASSESSMENT

A. Prognostic factors, Patient-related

➢ **General condition of the patient** and associated diseases

➢ **Extremes of age** (too old or too young) have poor prognosis

➢ **Gender**: male breast cancer has poor prognosis

➢ **Local complications**: intestinal obstruction or perforation in colorectal carcinoma, portal vein obstruction in HCC

➢ **High levels of tumour markers** pre-operative, e.g., CEA in colon cancer

B. Prognostic factors, Tumour-related

MACROSCOPIC:

➢ *Stage (single most important prognostic factor):* This depends on presence/absence of distant metastasis, tumour size and depth of invasion. Blood spread is worse than lymphatic spread. Two types of staging; *Pathological* staging and *Clinical* staging. Staging systems include TNM, AJCC, FIGO (gynaecologic tumours) Ann Arbor (lymphoma) and Duke's (colon, not used now).

➢ *Tumour site:* tumours in vital organs carry a worse prognosis

➢ *Tumour size:* the larger the size, the more the capacity of the tumour to metastasise

➢ *Tumour multiplicity:* has worse prognosis, especially seen in biliary and urinary tract cancers which result in synchronous or metachronous tumours

> ➤ **Tumour shape:** exophytic (fungating, cauliflower-like) is better than ulcerated. The latter has a better prognosis than the diffuse infiltrating form (annular stenosing, circumferential growth)

MICROSCOPIC:

➤ **Histological Grade** *(undifferentiated tumours have worse prognosis)*. Grading is the microscopic assessment of tumour differentiation. Tumour differentiation is the degree of tumour similarity to the tissue of origin (no clinical grading).

1. **Cellular grading** depends on cellular atypia (including pleomorphism), number of mitosis, +/-necrosis as in Blooms-Richardson's scoring of breast carcinoma.
2. **Architectural grading** assesses the deviation of tumour units (e.g., acini) from the normal glandular pattern as in Gleason's scoring.
3. **Nuclear grading** evaluates the size and shape of the nucleus and nucleolus as in grading of renal cell carcinoma and uterine adenocarcinoma.

➤ **Tumour type:** Mucinous carcinoma of the GIT has worse prognosis than classical adenocarcinoma, while mucinous carcinoma of the breast has a better prognosis than conventional IDC of the breast.

➤ **Precancerous lesions:** hepatocellular carcinoma on top of cirrhosis has worse prognosis due to high recurrence rate

➤ **Tumour edge:** infiltrating edge is worse than pushing edge

➤ **Tumour budding:** the presence of single cells or few groups of cells at the tumour edge carries worse prognosis.

C. Prognostic factors, Treatment-related

➤ **Completeness of resection**: resected tumours with tumour-free safety margins have better prognosis

➤ **Recurrence after surgical resection** (bad): recurrence usually associated with high grade/stage

➤ **Chemo/radio-resistant tumours** have poor prognosis. Factors related to tumour resistance include bcl-2, heat shock proteins, multi-drug resistance (MDR) proteins

D. IHC prognostic markers:

Examples:

- CD56 negative myeloma has poor prognosis. CD56+ lymphocytes may be associated with regression of melanoma
- ER, PR and Her2 in breast carcinoma

E. Prognostic factors, Molecular assay

➤ Over expression, amplifications or increased number of oncogene copies have poor prognosis, e.g., EGF, N-Myc in neuroblastoma

➤ Mutations of cancer suppressor genes, e.g., BRCA-1, p53 mutations generally associated with poor prognosis

➤ Receptor over expression or mutation, e.g., ER/PR or HER2-neu associated with poor prognosis

Mutations of signal transducers, e.g., K-Ras correlated with poor prognosis

➤ Absence of some genes or proteins linked with prognosis, e.g., nm23 (non-metastasis gene)

➤ Loss of E-cadherin in epithelial cancers associated with bad prognosis

➤ DNA aneuploidy by flow cytometry indicates an aggressive tumour

F. Prognostic factors, Tumour Behaviour

➤ **Invasion helpers/inhibitors**: balance between plasminogen activators/inhibitors, collagenases & metalloproteinases and their inhibitors and Cathepsin D determines the invasive capacity

➤ **Tumour cell proliferation rate** measured by mitotic count/ 10 hpf, Ki-67 staining, S-phase by flow cytometry or Bromodeoxyuridine labelling

➤ **Lymphatic-vascular invasion:** if present, poorer prognosis

➤ **Increased tumour angiogenesis** assessed by micro-vessel density or vascular endothelial growth factor (VEGF) staining

➤ **Production of high levels of blood group antigens, insulin-like growth factor, prostate-specific antigen**

MISMATCH REPAIR (MICROSATELLITE INSTABILITY, MSI) TESTING IN COLORECTAL CANCER (CRC) AND ENDOMETRIAL CANCER

MLH1, MSH2, MSH6 and PMS2 IHC are performed (panel of 4)

MMR-deficient = MMR germ line mutation (Lynch syndrome, MSI+), 14% of all CRC tumours = better prognosis, less metastasis

Pathological features in CRC: mucinous differentiation or solid + excess tumour-infiltrating lymphocytes (Medullary-like).

Clinical features: <50 y, proximal tumours

Internal control: Background stromal cells showed strong positive nuclear staining for the above antibodies.

Normal pattern (MMR proficient gene), the tumour expresses the following:

MLH1 - Strong and diffuse nuclear positivity.
MSH2 - Strong and diffuse nuclear positivity.
MSH6 - Strong and diffuse nuclear positivity.
PMS2 - Strong and diffuse nuclear positivity.

Reference values
1. Normal Pattern (MMR proficient): MLH1+, MSH2+, MSH6+, PMS2+
2. MMR gene mutations (MMR deficient, Lynch syndrome):
   - MLH1 Gene: stains: MLH1-, MSH2+, MSH6+, PMS2-
   - MSH2 Gene: stains: MLH1+, MSH2-, MSH6-, PMS2+
   - MSH6 Gene: stains: MLH1+, MSH2+, MSH6-, PMS2+
   - PMS2 Gene: stains: MLH1+, MSH2+, MSH6+, PMS2-

INTERPRETATION:
- A tumour that is MLH1- and PMS2- = MMR loss= sporadic MSI cancer
- A tumour that is MSH2- and MSH6- = germline mutation

REFERENCES

1.   EZTNM for the AJCC cancer staging manual. 2003, Springer-Verlag: New York. p. 1 CD-ROM.
2.   EZTNM for the AJCC cancer staging manual. 2003, Springer-Verlag: New York. p. 1 CD-ROM.
3.   Agnes, A., et al., Global updates in the treatment of gastric cancer: a systematic review. Part 1: staging, classification and surgical treatment. Updates Surg. 72(2): p. 341-353.
4.   Alghamdi, A.O., et al., Low grade appendiceal mucinous neoplasm mimicking an ovarian cyst: A case report. Int J Surg Case Rep. 70: p. 145-148.
5.   AlHammad, F., et al., Eyelid sebaceous gland carcinoma: An assessment of the T classification of the American Joint Committee of Cancer TNM staging system 8th versus 7th edition. Eur J Ophthalmol: p. 1120672120936488.
6.   Aljabab, S., et al., Proton Therapy for Locally Advanced Oropharyngeal Cancer: Initial Clinical Experience at the University of Washington. Int J Part Ther. 6(3): p. 1-12.
7.   Almangush, A., et al., Staging and grading of oral squamous cell carcinoma: An update. Oral Oncol. 107: p. 104799.
8.   Almangush, A., et al., Risk stratification in oral squamous cell carcinoma using staging of the eighth American Joint Committee on Cancer: Systematic review and meta-analysis. Head Neck.
9.   Amaral, T.M.S., et al., Clinical validation of a prognostic 11-gene expression profiling score in prospectively collected FFPE tissue of patients with AJCC v8 stage II cutaneous melanoma. Eur J Cancer. 125: p. 38-45.
10.   Amin, M.B., American Joint Committee on Cancer., and American Cancer Society., AJCC cancer staging manual. Eight edition / editor-in-chief, Mahul B. Amin, MD, FCAP ; editors, Stephen B. Edge, MD, FACS [and 16 others] ; Donna M. Gress, RHIT, CTR - Technical editor ; Laura R. Meyer, CAPM - Managing editor. ed. xvii, 1024 pages.
11.   Amin, M.B., American Joint Committee on Cancer., and American Cancer Society., AJCC cancer staging manual. Eight edition / editor-in-chief, Mahul B. Amin, MD, FCAP ; editors, Stephen B. Edge, MD, FACS [and 16 others] ; Donna M. Gress, RHIT, CTR - Technical editor ; Laura R. Meyer, CAPM - Managing editor. ed. xvii, 1024 pages.
12.   Ammori, B.J., Re: Modified Gastric Cancer AJCC Staging with a Classification Based on the Ratio of Regional Lymph Node Involvement: A Population-Based Cohort Study. Ann Surg Oncol.
13.   Arabiki, M., et al., Verification of the Japanese staging system for rectal cancer, focusing on differences with the TNM classification. Surg Today.
14.   Aygun, N. and M. Uludag, Pheochromocytoma and Paraganglioma: From Epidemiology to Clinical Findings. Sisli Etfal Hastan Tip Bul. 54(2): p. 159-168.
15.   Baba, A., et al., Radiological approach for the newly incorporated T staging factor, depth of invasion (DOI), of the oral tongue cancer in the 8th edition of American Joint Committee on Cancer (AJCC) staging manual: assessment of the necessity for elective neck dissection. Jpn J Radiol.
16.   Bajaj, S., et al., Melanoma Prognosis - Accuracy of the American Joint Committee on Cancer Staging Manual Eighth Edition. J Natl Cancer Inst.
17.   Bando, E., et al., Development and validation of a pretreatment nomogram to predict overall survival in gastric cancer. Cancer Med.
18.   Bauer, E., et al., Extranodal extension is a strong prognosticator in HPV-positive oropharyngeal squamous cell carcinoma. Laryngoscope. 130(4): p. 939-945.
19.   Berry, D.E., et al., Correlation of Gene Expression Profile Status and American Joint Commission on Cancer Stage in Uveal Melanoma. Retina. 40(2): p. 214-224.
20.   Chan, E.G., et al., Outcomes with segmentectomy versus lobectomy in patients with clinical T1cN0M0 non-small cell lung cancer. J Thorac Cardiovasc Surg.

21.   Chandramohan, A., et al., Diffusion weighted imaging improves diagnostic ability of MRI for determining complete response to neoadjuvant therapy in locally advanced rectal cancer. Eur J Radiol Open. 7: p. 100223.

22.   Chawla, A., et al., Clinical staging in pancreatic adenocarcinoma underestimates extent of disease. Pancreatology. 20(4): p. 691-697.

23.   Chen, C.Y., et al., Prognostic Value of Tumor Size in Resected Stage IIIA-N2 Non-Small-Cell Lung Cancer. J Clin Med. 9(5).

24.   Chen, Q.Y., et al., Conditional survival and recurrence of remnant gastric cancer after surgical resection: A multi-institutional study. Cancer Sci. 111(2): p. 502-512.

25.   Chen, Y.J., et al., A reappraisal of lymph node dissection in colorectal cancer during primary surgical resection. World J Surg Oncol. 18(1): p. 97.

26.   Chen, Z., et al., Marital status independently predicts non-small cell lung cancer survival: a propensity-adjusted SEER database analysis. J Cancer Res Clin Oncol. 146(1): p. 67-74.

27.   Chuang, S.T., et al., Tumor histologic grade as a risk factor for neck recurrence in patients with T1-2N0 early tongue cancer. Oral Oncol. 106: p. 104706.

28.   Comperat, E., et al., Dataset for the reporting of carcinoma of the bladder-cystectomy, cystoprostatectomy and diverticulectomy specimens: recommendations from the International Collaboration on Cancer Reporting (ICCR). Virchows Arch. 476(4): p. 521-534.

29.   Compton, C.C. and American Joint Committee on Cancer., AJCC cancer staging atlas : a companion to the seventh editions of the AJCC cancer staging manual and handbook. Second edition / ed. xi, 637 pages.

30.   Compton, C.C. and American Joint Committee on Cancer., AJCC cancer staging atlas : a companion to the seventh editions of the AJCC cancer staging manual and handbook. Second edition / ed. xi, 637 pages.

31.   Compton, M.L. and J.M.M. Cates, Evidence-based Tumor Staging of Skeletal Chondrosarcoma. Am J Surg Pathol. 44(1): p. 111-119.

32.   Cornejo, K.M., T. Rice-Stitt, and C.L. Wu, Updates in Staging and Reporting of Genitourinary Malignancies. Arch Pathol Lab Med. 144(3): p. 305-319.

33.   Cui, C., et al., Machine Learning Analysis of Image Data Based on Detailed MR Image Reports for Nasopharyngeal Carcinoma Prognosis. Biomed Res Int. 2020: p. 8068913.

34.   Dang, Y., et al., Clinical complete regression after local radiotherapy combined with chemotherapy for stage IV rectal cancer: A case report. Mol Clin Oncol. 13(2): p. 186-190.

35.   Davis, R.J., et al., From presumed benign neck masses to delayed recognition of human papillomavirus-positive oropharyngeal cancer. Laryngoscope. 130(2): p. 392-397.

36.   Deng, B.Y., et al., Survivals of patients with pancreatic neuroendocrine carcinomas: An in-depth analysis by the American Joint Committee on Cancer 8th tumor-node-metastasis staging manual. Medicine (Baltimore). 99(3): p. e18736.

37.   Deng, J., et al., Relationship between T stage and survival in distantly metastatic esophageal cancer: A STROBE-compliant study. Medicine (Baltimore). 99(19): p. e20064.

38.   Deng, Y., et al., Magnetic resonance imaging for preoperative staging of pancreatic cancer based on the 8(th) edition of AJCC guidelines. J Gastrointest Oncol. 11(2): p. 329-336.

39.   Dhar, H., R. Vaish, and A.K. D'Cruz, Management of locally advanced oral cancers. Oral Oncol. 105: p. 104662.

40.   D'Ugo, D., et al., Global updates in the treatment of gastric cancer: a systematic review. Part 2: perioperative management, multimodal therapies, new technologies, standardization of the surgical treatment and educational aspects. Updates Surg. 72(2): p. 355-378.

41.   Edge, S.B. and American Joint Committee on Cancer., AJCC cancer staging manual. 7th ed, New York: Springer. xiv, 648 p.

42.   Edge, S.B. and American Joint Committee on Cancer., AJCC cancer staging manual. 7th ed, New York: Springer. xiv, 648 p.

43.   Edge, S.B., American Joint Committee on Cancer., and American Cancer Society., AJCC cancer staging handbook : from the AJCC cancer staging manual. 7th ed, New York: Springer. xix, 718 p.

44.	Edge, S.B., American Joint Committee on Cancer., and American Cancer Society., AJCC cancer staging handbook : from the AJCC cancer staging manual. 7th ed, New York: Springer. xix, 718 p.
45.	Elias, M.L., et al., Localized Sebaceous Carcinoma Treatment: Wide Local Excision verses Mohs Micrographic Surgery. Dermatol Ther: p. e13991.
46.	Ellis, R., et al., Epidermal autophagy and beclin 1 regulator 1 and loricrin: a paradigm shift in the prognostication and stratification of the American Joint Committee on Cancer stage I melanomas. Br J Dermatol. 182(1): p. 156-165.
47.	Fagan, J.J., et al., Is AJCC/UICC Staging Still Appropriate for Head and Neck Cancers in Developing Countries? OTO Open. 4(3): p. 2473974X20938313.
48.	Farley, C.R., et al., Merkel Cell Carcinoma Outcomes: Does AJCC8 Underestimate Survival? Ann Surg Oncol. 27(6): p. 1978-1985.
49.	Farquhar, D.R., et al., Evaluation of pathologic staging using number of nodes in p16-negative head and neck cancer. Oral Oncol. 108: p. 104800.
50.	Felismino, T.C., et al., Primary Tumor Location Is a Predictor of Poor Prognosis in Patients with Locally Advanced Esophagogastric Cancer Treated with Perioperative Chemotherapy. J Gastrointest Cancer. 51(2): p. 484-490.
51.	Fleming, I.D., et al., AJCC cancer staging manual. 5th ed / ed. 1997, Philadelphia: Lippincott-Raven. xv, 294 p.
52.	Fleming, I.D., et al., AJCC cancer staging manual. 5th ed / ed. 1997, Philadelphia: Lippincott-Raven. xv, 294 p.
53.	Flukes, S., et al., Primary tumor volume as a predictor of distant metastases and survival in patients with sinonasal mucosal melanoma. Head Neck.
54.	Foo, C.C., et al., How does lymph node yield affect survival outcomes of stage I and II colon cancer? World J Surg Oncol. 18(1): p. 22.
55.	Freitag, J., et al., Extracapsular extension of neck nodes and absence of human papillomavirus 16-DNA are predictors of impaired survival in p16-positive oropharyngeal squamous cell carcinoma. Cancer. 126(9): p. 1856-1872.
56.	Gaspersz, M.P., et al., Evaluation of the New American Joint Committee on Cancer Staging Manual 8th Edition for Perihilar Cholangiocarcinoma. J Gastrointest Surg. 24(7): p. 1612-1618.
57.	Ge, D., et al., Development and Validation of a Nomogram-Based Prognostic Evaluation Model for Sarcomatoid Hepatocellular Carcinoma. Adv Ther. 37(7): p. 3185-3205.
58.	Geng, Y., et al., Identification of m6A-related genes and m6A RNA methylation regulators in pancreatic cancer and their association with survival. Ann Transl Med. 8(6): p. 387.
59.	Glastonbury, C.M., Head and Neck Squamous Cell Cancer: Approach to Staging and Surveillance. p. 215-222.
60.	Gomez-Acebo, I., et al., Tumour characteristics and survivorship in a cohort of breast cancer: the MCC-Spain study. Breast Cancer Res Treat. 181(3): p. 667-678.
61.	Gong, Y., et al., A novel lymph node staging system for gastric cancer including modified Union for cancer Control/American Joint Committee on cancer and Japanese Gastric Cancer Association criteria. Eur J Surg Oncol.
62.	Greene, F.L. and American Joint Committee on Cancer., AJCC cancer staging atlas. 2006, New York, NY: Springer. ix, 352 p.
63.	Greene, F.L. and American Joint Committee on Cancer., AJCC cancer staging atlas. 2006, New York, NY: Springer. ix, 352 p.
64.	Greene, F.L., American Joint Committee on Cancer., and American Cancer Society., AJCC cancer staging handbook : from the AJCC cancer staging manual. 6th ed. 2002, New York: Springer. xv, 469 p.
65.	Greene, F.L., American Joint Committee on Cancer., and American Cancer Society., AJCC cancer staging manual. 6th ed. 2002, New York: Springer-Verlag. xiv, 421 p.
66.	Greene, F.L., American Joint Committee on Cancer., and American Cancer Society., AJCC cancer staging handbook : from the AJCC cancer staging manual. 6th ed. 2002, New York: Springer. xv, 469 p.

67.   Greene, F.L., American Joint Committee on Cancer., and American Cancer Society., AJCC cancer staging manual. 6th ed. 2002, New York: Springer-Verlag. xiv, 421 p.

68.   Gu, L., et al., The relationship between the number of examined lymph nodes and the efficacy of chemotherapy for gastric cancer. Surg Today. 50(6): p. 585-596.

69.   Gulmez, S., et al., The prognostic value of different lymph node classification systems in stage III colorectal cancer patients. Ann Ital Chir. 9.

70.   Hahn, F., et al., Risk prediction in intrahepatic cholangiocarcinoma: Direct comparison of the MEGNA score and the 8th edition of the UICC/AJCC Cancer staging system. PLoS One. 15(2): p. e0228501.

71.   Haider, S.P., et al., Potential Added Value of PET/CT Radiomics for Survival Prognostication beyond AJCC 8th Edition Staging in Oropharyngeal Squamous Cell Carcinoma. Cancers (Basel). 12(7).

72.   Han, J., et al., Reassessment of American Joint Committee on Cancer Staging for Stage III Renal Cell Carcinoma With Nodal Involvement: Propensity Score Matched Analyses of a Large Population-Based Study. Front Oncol. 10: p. 365.

73.   Han, L., et al., Comparison of four lymph node staging systems for predicting prognosis for stage IV rectum cancer. Ann Transl Med. 8(4): p. 111.

74.   Han, L., et al., Prognostic accuracy of different lymph node staging system in predicting overall survival in stage IV colon cancer. Int J Colorectal Dis. 35(2): p. 317-322.

75.   Hank, T., et al., A Combination of Biochemical and Pathological Parameters Improves Prediction of Postresection Survival After Preoperative Chemotherapy in Pancreatic Cancer: The PANAMA-score. Ann Surg.

76.   He, J., et al., AJCC 8th edition prognostic staging provides no better discriminatory ability in prognosis than anatomical staging in triple negative breast cancer. BMC Cancer. 20(1): p. 18.

77.   Hieken, T.J., et al., Sex-Based Differences in Melanoma Survival in a Contemporary Patient Cohort. J Womens Health (Larchmt).

78.   Hirshoren, N., J.M. Weinberger, and R. Eliashar, [Head and Neck Malignancies Classification, the 8th Edition of the American Joint Committee on Cancer - What Is New?]. Harefuah. 159(1): p. 132-136.

79.   Hong, T., et al., Development and validation of a nomogram to predict survival after curative resection of nonmetastatic colorectal cancer. Cancer Med. 9(12): p. 4126-4136.

80.   Hu, D., et al., Is a simplified TNM staging system more clinically relevant than the American Joint Committee on Cancer system for the follicular variant of papillary thyroid cancer? Ann Transl Med. 8(7): p. 463.

81.   Hu, J., et al., Improved Prognostication for the Updated AJCC Breast Cancer Pathological Prognostic Staging Varied in Higher-Stage Groups. Clin Breast Cancer. 20(3): p. 253-261 e7.

82.   Hu, P., et al., Trends of incidence and prognosis of gastric neuroendocrine neoplasms: a study based on SEER and our multicenter research. Gastric Cancer. 23(4): p. 591-599.

Index

A

Adenocarcinoma, 29, 41
ADENOCARCINOMA, 66
ADENOID CYSTIC CARCINOMA, 67
Adenosarcoma, 42
Adrenal Cortical Carcinoma, 46
AJCC, 13, 82, 87, 88, 89, 90
Ampulla of Vater, 28
Anal canal, 30
angiogenesis, 6, 43, 85
Appendix, 29, 58
APPENDIX, 32
ASTROCYTIC TUMOURS, 74

B

bile ducts, 34, 35, 79
BONE TUMOURS, 49
breast. *See*
BREAST, 38, 71, 76

C

Carcinoma in situ, 15
Carcinoma of Skin of the Eyelid, 54
CARCINOMA OF UNKNOWN PRIMARY, 24
carcinosarcoma, 41
CERVICAL INTRAEPITHELIAL NEOPLSIA, 69
Cervix, 13, 41
chondrosarcoma, 49
collagenase, 6, 7
COLON, 33
Colon-Rectum, 29
Conjunctival carcinoma, 54
Cribriform, 67

D

DCIS, 3, 15, 38, 66, 76, 77
Depth of invasion, 3, 16, 20, 31, 40

DOI, 3, 15, 16, 20, 22, 40, 41, 87
DUCTAL CARCINOMA IN SITU, 71

E

ECE, 22
EFFECT OF LOCAL/DIRECT TUMOUR SPREAD, 11
EMVI, 3, 29
Endometrioid adenocarcinoma, 69
ENE, 3, 17, 23, 26, 40, 45, 51
Ewing, 49, 59, 75

F

Fallopian tube, 42
FIGO, 10, 13, 40, 41, 42, 43, 60, 82
FNCLCC grading system, 75
Fuhrman grading, 73

G

Gall bladder, 19, 35
Gestational Trophoblastic Tumours, 42
GIST, 31, 48
GLEASON GRADING, 68
Glottis, 24
Grade, 31, 32, 43, 45, 46, 49, 66, 69, 71, 73, 74, 75, 77, 79, 83

H

HAEMATOGENOUS (BLOOD) SPREAD, 9
Haggitt, 63
Head & neck, 22
HEAD AND NECK, 22
hepatoblastoma, 59, 60, 61
Hepatoblastoma, 59
HEPATOCELLULAR CARCINOMA, 73
HOLLOW ORGANS, 11
HPV, 23, 24, 26, 41, 45, 69, 87

www.ingramcontent.com/pod-product-compliance
Lightning Source LLC
Chambersburg PA
CBHW051220170526
45166CB00005B/1973